The Other Mothers

The Other Mothers

TWO WOMEN'S JOURNEY TO FIND THE
FAMILY THAT WAS ALWAYS THEIRS

Jennifer Berney

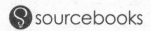

Published by Sourcebooks
P.O. Box 4410, Naperville, Illinois 60567-4410
(630) 961-3900
sourcebooks.com

Library of Congress Cataloging-in-Publication Data

Names: Berney, Jennifer (Creative writing teacher), author.
Title: The other mothers : two women's journey to find the family that was
   always theirs / Jennifer Berney.
Description: Naperville : Sourcebooks, 2021. | Includes bibliographical
   references.
Identifiers: LCCN 2020035770 (print) | LCCN 2020035771 (ebook) |
Subjects: LCSH: Lesbian mothers--United States. | Families--United States.
   | Sexual orientation--United States. | Artificial insemination,
   Human--United States.
Classification: LCC HQ75.53 .B47 2021 (print) | LCC HQ75.53 (ebook) | DDC
   306.874/3086643--dc23
LC record available at https://lccn.loc.gov/2020035770
LC ebook record available at https://lccn.loc.gov/2020035771

Printed and bound in the United States of America.
VP 10 9 8 7 6 5 4 3 2 1

To my family

CONTENTS

I.

PROLOGUE

I was twelve years old when I first heard the term test-tube baby—when my brain, for the first time, reckoned with the idea that doctors and outsiders could have a hand in conception, that one man and one woman sharing a bed was not the only way to make a child.

I heard the term *test-tube baby* while sitting cross-legged on the floor of my fifth-grade classroom. That year was my first at a small Quaker school where we called our teachers by their first names, held silent worship every Tuesday, and learned things they didn't teach in public school. We read books on civil rights, studied the history of nuclear armament, and sang songs by Pete Seeger. It was the year I cut my bangs too short and wore a painter's cap to hide them, the year I checked for new zits each time I looked in the mirror, the year that I looked on as boys and girls began to pair off with each other. It was the year that after lunch on Wednesdays, our teachers gathered us in a circle to teach us about sex and the human body.

In my memory, the scene unfolds like this:

Helen, one of our teachers, stands at the front of the class and lectures about reproduction. She's a short, round woman with kind eyes and a head of untamed black curls. There are times when Helen is casual and fun, but today she is all business; she wears a collared shirt and points at the board with a fresh piece of chalk. She uses words we've already learned from xeroxed handouts: *testicles, vas deferens, urethra, ovary, ovum, follicle.* She uses the words *penis* and *vagina.* She is talking about sex. She calls it *intercourse.* We know better than to laugh. Laughter would invite a lecture on how all parts of the body are natural and fine. We'd prefer that Helen moves on as quickly as possible.

Helen moves on. She asks what we know about other methods of conception. Other methods. We continue our stunned silence for a moment, until one boy raises his hand and blurts out, "Test-tube babies!" The class erupts in laughter, not so much because it's funny but because we've been holding our composure, and he has given us an opportunity to let it go. And, really, it is a little funny: the idea of babies popping out of test tubes.

Helen is patient. She waits for us to settle. She may even be hiding a smile. She proceeds to correct his language, to clarify that he's referring to *in vitro fertilization*, that the process happens in a lab with microscopes and petri dishes, not actual test tubes, that an embryo is created outside of the body and then introduced to a mother's womb. Maybe she goes on to discuss other modes of assisted reproduction, but I don't know because the scene fades out for me right there.

What remains is the phrase "test-tube baby," which became an image that lingered in my memory for years, like a thing I could reach out and grab.

At that time, I didn't learn anything about the original test-tube babies, like that they were conceived in Oldham, England, or that they were no longer babies but children. Louise Joy Brown, the very first test-tube baby, was conceived the same year I was born. The story of her conception goes like this: One day in November, Dr. Patrick Steptoe made an incision and, with a laparoscope, retrieved an egg from Mrs. Lesley Brown—a woman who, at only twenty-nine, had been trying to conceive for nearly a decade. Seven years earlier, she'd undergone surgery to treat blocked fallopian tubes, but her organs remained damaged and scarred.

Lesley Brown's husband John reported that their continued failure to conceive had pushed her into a severe depression and strained their marriage. Mr. Brown himself was veritably fertile, so while Dr. Steptoe retrieved the egg, a second doctor, Dr. Robert Edwards, prepared a sample of Mr. Brown's semen. With a pipette, a microscope, and a petri dish, Edwards introduced the sperm to the egg. He kept everything warm. He kept watch, waiting for the egg cell to cleave. Lesley Brown waited. Somewhere on the clinic grounds, among the dozens of other hopeful women undergoing similar treatments, she passed the hours. By the evening of the second day, cleavage had taken place. The egg had transformed into a two-celled zygote.

On the afternoon of the third day, Dr. Edwards and Dr. Steptoe waited some more, watching over the growing cluster of cells as daylight faded. There were two cells, then four, then six. They were waiting for eight—a number that indicated a viable embryo. This took time. Dr. Steptoe left for dinner. It was his wife's birthday, and they wanted to celebrate. When they returned, Dr. Edwards's wife had joined him at the clinic. Both couples sat together in the lab, talking into the night like kin, as the cells cleaved once more and became eight. They fetched Lesley Brown. It was after midnight then.

To place the embryo inside of Lesley Brown required no incision, only a cannula, syringe, and forceps. In expelling the embryo into her cervical canal, Dr. Edwards returned her egg transformed—not a single cell, but a living, growing thing. Together, these doctors accomplished in their lab what most often happens under blankets (or sometimes in an open field, or the back seat of a car).

If you read the firsthand accounts of this evening, you might conclude that though the Browns' conception was a clinical act, it was also a loving one. Jean Purdy, the nurse who worked doggedly alongside the doctors, returned Lesley Brown to her bed that night and reported that she whispered, "That was a wonderful experience."[1]

But other women who were part of the same experiment never conceived. These were women who had longed for a child so desperately that they spent weeks as inpatients, offering urine for testing every three hours. At night, they listened for the doctor, waiting to see if their door would be opened, if they would be summoned for egg retrieval.[2]

They had the same surgeries as Lesley Brown, the same procedures, and yet the embryos didn't take. In some cases, the doctors would later conclude, it was simply because they had introduced the embryo to the womb in the daytime, when adrenal hormone levels were higher, and ovarian hormones were lower.[3] These were women who were as determined and hopeful as Lesley Brown, but, because their wombs flushed away the embryo, because their periods arrived, we will never learn their names.

That day on the floor of my fifth-grade classroom, I didn't learn any of these details, but I thought a lot about the test tube and the possibilities it represented. I suspected I might someday make use of these possibilities. I suspected this because I worried I was different.

I was just starting to learn the language for this difference. In my memory, it was the same fifth-grade boy who blurted the answer "test-tube baby" who'd also leaned toward me one day at lunch and hissed, "Did you know that Helen is a lezzie?"

I didn't believe him. I didn't *not* believe him. Helen was Helen. I could not picture her with a husband, but then again, I'd never known any woman who had a wife. I could only picture her as our teacher, alone in front of the classroom. I shrugged away the rumor. But the word, *lezzie*, the seething disdain of it, struck me.

On another Wednesday, late in the school year, Helen invited two guests to our health and sexuality class. One was a gay man, the other a lesbian. They took turns introducing themselves and telling their stories. I studied them closely. The man had a crew cut and a turquoise sweater. The woman wore hoop earrings and an asymmetrical hairdo. When I looked at them, it seemed that I could spot their queerness—the hint that they played by a different set of rules—but what was more remarkable to me was that they also seemed normal, like people who might teach at my school or attend my mother's Unitarian church.

As I sat there, a small fear inside of me grew into a larger one. *What if I was like them?* I wondered. The thought panicked me because it struck me as possible. And even though they were there to provide evidence that they were real people who lived real lives, I felt a sense of dread: If I turned out to be gay, I believed my life would become unbearably small, that I might live alone in a dark apartment with one twin bed and a pile of books, with no friends or lovers to call on.

At some point, Helen asked the room for questions, and I raised my hand. "How do you know if you're gay?" I asked. It came out like a squeak. My face grew hot. All of the fifth-grade eyes were on me.

The lesbian looked at the gay man. She looked at me. "It takes a lot of soul-searching," she said.

The man nodded his head in agreement. I waited for them to explain, to offer some kind of criteria, a set of questions I could ask myself. Instead, they took the next question.

For the next many years of my life, from twelve to eighteen and beyond, I remembered the test-tube babies. I remembered that out there, beyond my world of immediate knowledge, there were possibilities for how to make a family, how to build a life that wasn't lonely. The science of fertility, as I'd imagined it, was benevolent and magic. It was a kind of magic I thought I might eventually need.

1

CERTAINTY

On the first morning of my honeymoon, I woke up next to Kellie, both of us naked under clean white sheets. Morning light burst through parted curtains. Outside, a brood of wild turkeys waddled down a hillside. They jabbered to each other and pecked at the lawn. Beyond that lawn was a two-lane highway, and beyond that highway was the ocean—I couldn't see or hear it, but I knew it was there. I pulled my knees to my chest. The world inside our cabin felt cocooned and still. I watched Kellie as she slept: her eyes closed, her nose pressed into the pillow, her left hand tucked beneath it. If I listened carefully, I could hear her breathing. I gazed at the stretch of smooth skin between her shoulders and the freckles below her collarbone. I wanted to touch her, but I didn't want to wake her.

We were married now, kind of, as married as two women could be. Yesterday—a thousand miles north in Olympia, Washington—we gathered friends and family in a circle on a lawn. We called it a wedding. We read vows, we traded rings and kissed, we cut a tiered cake whose frosting was melting in the sun, we drank red wine out of plastic cups. I wore a blue dress and, for the first time in years, lipstick. The outfit made me nervous. The wedding made me nervous. Months ago, I had tried to convince Kellie that we could marry each other by simply buying two rings and trading them in some memorable spot: a beach in Hawaii, the top of Mount Eleanor, our own backyard at sunset.

What did marriage mean to us anyways? I asked her. George W. Bush was our president then. Not a single U.S. state had challenged the Defense of Marriage Act—a federal law that explicitly forbade the recognition of same-sex unions. In my mind, marriage equality was a tiny black dot on a distant horizon, a destination that our people might arrive at in hundreds of years, long after my death. But on this day, our vows to each other would mean nothing to the state. When filling out official forms, we would continue to check the box that said *single*.

I wasn't sure I wanted folks to see me getting married-not-married. It felt make-believe, like inviting people to come and watch me throw a tea party for my stuffed animal collection. But Kellie didn't want a private ceremony. "I think that people are supposed to come and witness it," she told me. "I think that's kind of the point."

I didn't want her to be right, but I knew she was. "Okay," I agreed.

In the end, nearly everyone we invited came: Kellie's mother and stepfather, her father and his girlfriend, her two grandmothers who sat on folding chairs in the sun with their old lady hairdos, my parents, our brothers, our closest friends. They dressed up and bore gifts, and seemed, as far as I could tell, to think our union truly mattered.

Now, outside our honeymoon cabin, the turkeys moved on to some other hillside. Kellie's breathing stalled for a moment before she opened her eyes and stretched an arm toward the wall. I reached for her. Her skin was warm. I kissed her. She kissed me back.

"We're married now," I said. The declaration made me nervous once I said it. I wanted to amend it, to add an addendum. Instead, I held my breath.

"We are," Kellie said.

There was another thing I wanted to say, a question that sat there, always, nestled like an egg in the hollow of my ribcage. I opened my mouth and spoke it. "When should we have a baby?"

I had asked Kellie this before. Her answers were always evasive. "I don't like the idea of buying sperm," she had said once, or, another time: "That's going to be an awful lot of work." Still, I kept asking, hoping that one day she'd look me square in the eye and say, "Soon."

But Kellie didn't meet my eyes right away. She ran a finger along the inside edge of her ear like she was pushing at an itch.

Then she answered with another question: "Are you sure you want that?"

"I'm sure," I said. We both already knew this was true.

———————————

From birth to age seven, I was an only child. I didn't want to be. Our family home in a small suburb of Boston was cavernous—two stories of rooms with floors that creaked and windows that were painted shut. My own bedroom was gray with a crack that ran through the wall beside my bed. Sometimes, if I couldn't sleep, I studied it. On full-moon nights, light beamed through the giant backyard tree and cast strange shadows on the wall.

I longed for the brighter, louder homes of my neighborhood friends. My friend Alice lived on the bottom floor of a two-family house one street over from me. To get to her, I cut through the neighbor's backyard. Alice's parents were both artists, and the walls were covered with sketches. The house smelled like unfamiliar foods, like lentil soup and pesto. She had a sister and a cat named Oreo who spread out on the floor in the sunshine and purred when anyone came near.

And then there was Mandy Filcher's house—a white house with black shutters at the end of my block—where her mother lay in the backyard with her bikini top unfastened in the back. She had two older brothers and a room filled with Barbies. At Mandy's house, we ate Chips Ahoy! cookies and stole her mother's cans of Diet Tab. Throughout the day, all the neighborhood boys congregated outside. They rode bikes and played street hockey. They came in and brought snacks upstairs so they could eat while they played Atari.

My house wasn't like that. If I went looking for snacks in my cupboard, I'd be lucky to find a few dry crackers wrapped in cellophane. My father had his own cupboard where he kept a bag of Fritos, but if I wanted some, I had to ask him first. My mother took naps daily and cried sometimes. She was battling anxiety and depression, conditions I didn't understand, but experienced as a thickness in the air that filled our home. My father hated noise. "Shhhh," I instructed my friends if they came over.

I did have three half siblings, my father's children from a previous marriage. They were all nearly grown-up when my parents wed, and they lived in other states, but when they came to visit, my heart filled. They played games with me and listened to records.

Every day I daydreamed about how the house might change if I had a younger sibling crawling from room to room, filling the house with living sounds.

I lobbied for a baby. At bedtime, when I visited my mom in her bed, I told her I wouldn't care if it were a sister or brother. I'd love the baby no matter what. At the dinner table, I hounded both of my parents for an answer, saying, "So is it *yes* or is it *no* or is it *maybe?*"

My mother and father took turns answering, and the answer

was always "we'll see." I didn't realize that behind closed doors, my parents were having the same conversation. My mother wanted another child too.

One day in early autumn, my mother sought me out in our backyard, where I was soliciting affection from a neighborhood cat. "I have something to tell you," she said.

I didn't shout or clap my hands or leap for joy. I just stayed there in the grass and felt a tingle in my belly—the joy of expectation. It settled there and grew.

Some children beg for a sibling and when he arrives, they beg to send him back. I didn't. When my brother arrived, I bottle-fed him, spoon-fed him, cradled him, read to him, and sang him lullabies. On Saturday mornings, when he woke before my parents, I tiptoed into his room. My brother would reach for me as I unlatched the crib gate. I lifted him and carried him downstairs. He sat on my lap while I watched Saturday morning cartoons. Together, we ate dry Cheerios from a plastic bowl.

The biggest comfort of my childhood was this: for the remainder of my years at home, I had another body, smaller than mine, to care for.

As I grew older, my vision of a future family evolved. I dreamed of a partner who adored me, of a child I would love, of a home that felt comfortable and bright. I longed for this future life just as fervently as I nursed the fear that no one would ever want me.

My first girlfriend was a leather-wearing butch with bleach-blond hair. I was eighteen and still in high school. She was twenty-three, a grown-up who paid her own rent and lived with roommates who worked day jobs. My teenage acne had mostly faded. My hair had grown long. On most days I could look in the mirror without wanting to hide my face behind a paper bag. Still, I was stunned that she had chosen me—that anyone had. I had spent years preparing myself for the possibility that I might die a virgin. "Sleep over tonight," she had said on the evening of our third date. Within two weeks, I was spending most of my nights at her apartment, in her bed. My skin was raw from her touch; everything inside of me was bursting. My body, it suddenly seemed, could not be contained.

It was spring in Boston. Trails of pollen floated on the surface of puddles. Magnolia buds burst and fell; rain drenched them; feet crushed them into the sidewalk. The air was still thick with that rain and that smell, which entered my girlfriend's apartment through an open window. Her roommates sat on the couch watching TV and smoking cigarettes while she sat in the armchair, and I sat in her lap. She whispered a secret: "I love you."

I wanted a baby right then, wanted to grow something inside of me, wanted to push it out, to break open, to welcome some tiny thing, crying and unfurling.

And then one evening, as I sat bare-legged on her mattress on the floor, she said, "I want to be honest with you." She told me about Cassie, another eighteen-year-old who worked beside her all day at the deli. I had seen Cassie before. She had light-brown hair that grew well past her waist and wore cut-off shorts that revealed her smooth thighs. She was tall and lanky with crooked teeth, and her beauty was extra striking because it seemed unintentional. My girlfriend told me about a conversation they'd had that day, inside the walk-in cooler. "I'm in a relationship," my girlfriend had told her. "But I just want you to know that I like you."

"I like you too," Cassie had said in return.

I sat there pinching the seam of the mattress between my fingers, waiting to hear if there was more.

"I just want to be honest. I don't want you to be jealous."

"I'm not jealous," I said. My throat swelled and burned. That night as she slept, I looked out her window and watched a seagull fly across the dark sky. It was one night of many nights that I wondered what love was supposed to feel like. I wondered if it was supposed to be so painful, to leave me feeling confused and open and raw, like a mussel dropped from the sky to the sidewalk, cracked and orange and exposed.

I couldn't answer those questions for myself, and so I stayed with her for four more years. We moved across the country together, from Boston to Seattle, from a landscape of deciduous trees and rolling hills to one of evergreens and mountains. One afternoon, alone in the apartment we shared, my first girlfriend declared that she was ready for a baby. "I want you to carry it," she told me. She put a hand on my waist when she said it and slid her hand underneath the hem of my shirt to touch my skin. I cringed. She never touched me anymore unless she wanted something. Lately she had taken to making schedules that laid out, day by day, who did what chores and who made what for dinner. I obeyed her charts, but still she complained that I didn't meet her standards. The dinner was too salty; the dishes hadn't been stacked the way she preferred them.

"I don't know," was the only answer I could manage. But the truth was that I did know. I didn't want a baby—not with her. Instead, I dreamed of a child with some unknown future partner. My imagined child was a comfort to me, a certainty. Its presence kept me company. That's what parenthood meant to me—that someday my loneliness would be interrupted.

I was twenty-two when I left, and I landed in a one-room apartment in a building populated by other single women. The windows in my new home reached from the floor to the ceiling; the space was always bright. There was a place for my bed and a place for my books and a closet for my clothes. I had two cats and one houseplant that I tended. The first night I spent there, I marveled at the quiet. I made myself dinner. I put the dishes in the sink. I played music and set the volume exactly where I wanted it. No one complained about the CD I had chosen or that I'd overcooked the spaghetti. No one asked me when I was planning to get to those dishes.

After a week of living like this, I discovered that I was

reliable. I could take care of myself, my cats, and my plant, and still I had giving left to spare. This room in me became a space for longing. I imagined a love that wasn't painful and a family built around that love.

I had slept alone every night for over a year on the day that Kellie walked into the neighborhood bakery where I worked. I had seen her there before—she came in weekly, but for some reason, on that day I took notice. She was in her thirties, taller than me, and kept her hair tied back in a ponytail that was forever coming loose. She had strong features, but there was also something soft about her: she wore Carhartt pants with worn-out T-shirts and drove an old Ford pickup with a dog in the passenger's seat. When she pulled up and parked in front of the bakery, her dog moved to the driver's side and panted, waiting intently while Kellie came in. She asked for a cup of coffee, and I poured her one. Our eyes didn't lock. The sky didn't fall. But on my way to sleep that night, I remembered her face and thought, *If I were ten years older, that's exactly who I'd want.* Maybe, when I too was in my thirties, I would find someone exactly like that, someone with long hair and cool blue eyes, someone kind with just the right amount of swagger.

Four months later I heard someone call out "Hey!" in a grocery store parking lot. It was Kellie, getting ready to climb in her truck. "It's my favorite bakery girl," she said.

"Hey," I called back, extracting a hand from deep in my coat pocket to wave. It was four thirty in the afternoon, and, because it was late December, the sun was already sinking toward the horizon, blazing a clear, winter orange. I was headed toward the sidewalk, preparing to walk home alone.

"Happy New Year!" she called out.

"Happy New Year!" I called back.

I thought of her the whole way home as I walked down a long hill and watched the sky fade to twilight, and then once I was home I thought about her some more. I was surprised that someone had noticed me. I lived in Olympia, Washington, home of Evergreen State College and the Riot Grrrl movement. If Seattle was Washington's heart, then Olympia was its armpit. Our grunge was grungier, our rainy days were rainier, and our queers were queerer. The lesbians around town sported tattoos and piercings, pink hair and fishnets. I wanted to be like them, but I wasn't. With my ponytail and sensible shoes, I looked like someone's out-of-town cousin—the kind of person you'd meet at a party and instantly forget.

But Kellie, for whatever reason, noticed me. I thought of her every day at the bakery, my whole body poised for her appearance from the moment we opened at six in the morning until the moment I left at one in the afternoon. When she did come in, we never chatted, but it seemed that she leaned into the counter as she ordered, and I felt a wild electricity run through me. By then it had become clear to me that I didn't care about the age gap that separated us: I didn't want Kellie's equivalent in ten years; I wanted the actual Kellie, now.

One day at the bakery, Kellie overheard me explaining to a coworker that I still didn't have a driver's license. Not driving was a point of angst for me. I had wanted to learn as a teenager, but my mother had declared that she was too anxious to teach me, and my father, though willing, winced each time I turned a corner. His tension fed my own. I lacked the kind of teenage bravado that would have allowed me to steal the keys in the middle of the night. Soon enough I was seventeen without a license, and then eighteen, and then nineteen, and with each year the task of learning to drive began to seem more and more impossible.

Now, as a twentysomething in Olympia, I got by okay without a car or license. I took the bus to school, walked to the grocery store, and biked to work. When my cats needed to go to the vet, I called a cab. But I felt embarrassed that I couldn't, for instance, drive myself to a nearby mountain for a day hike or go for a road trip with friends and trade off at the wheel. Not driving made me feel dependent and vulnerable, stuck in a teenage fear.

Kellie approached the counter. "I can teach you to drive," she said. She grabbed an order slip from the counter and wrote down her name and phone number. I'd later understand that this was exactly how Kellie made all of her connections: by listening for a need that she might fill. Maybe someone was looking for a chainsaw to borrow or needed a hand figuring out why their dryer wasn't working. Kellie was there for that, and as a result she had a vast network of friends and acquaintances all over town who knew her as someone who could take care of things. I was in awe of her. I knew nothing about chainsaws or dryers, but I wanted to know everything about her.

We drove together on Sundays, on back roads—roads I'd never seen for the simple reason that I didn't have a car. They were roads that brought you nowhere in particular, roads that wove through mossy forests, up and down gentle slopes, occasionally revealing a distant peek of Puget Sound or the snowy crest of Mount Rainier. Because it was spring, most Sundays brought all kinds of weather. We drove through storms that cleared to blinding light.

Kellie pretended it was no big deal for a near-stranger to take the wheel of her car, and so I pretended it was no big deal for me to drive. There was magic in that. I didn't want to embarrass myself by making sudden swerves or stops, and so I cruised along, exhilarated, feigning competence.

We talked about nothing in particular—about movies we liked and books we read, about places we'd lived and places we always wanted to go. As we spoke, I felt cloaked in a kind of rapt attention that I'd rarely received and always craved. "I think about you a lot," Kellie told me at the end of our third Sunday drive.

After the first night we spent together, Kellie joked, "I might have to marry you now." It was July, and we had slept in an outdoor bedroom she had assembled under a party tent in her

backyard. Kellie lived in a small bungalow her grandfather had
built in the 1920s, and she was in the midst of repainting the
walls and refinishing the floors. The night before, we had eaten
dinner at a makeshift table in the living room, but the bed, the
dressers, the bedside tables—those were all outside. The idea
of sleeping outside was romantic, but we were too nervous to
enjoy it. I spent most of the night awake, listening and waiting,
sensing the body that lay next to me, wondering if she was
sleeping. It seemed that I'd only been sleeping for moments
when dawn woke me. Birds called to each other from one tree
to the next. Our pillows and covers were now damp from the
morning air. Kellie was awake too. Something about morning's
arrival relaxed us. We found each other easily. By the time the
sun crested the hill, I was breathless and hushed. That's when
she said it. "I might have to marry you now." It was a joke but not
a joke. I laughed and leaned into her, yet I sensed that if I had
said, *Fine, let's do it*, she wouldn't have backed down.

One morning, about a week later, I woke to the sound of
pebbles being tossed against my window. My apartment building had no intercom, and so this was the most efficient way to
reach me. When I looked outside, it was Kellie, her head tilted
toward my second-story window. The sky behind her was
cloudless. "I called in sick at work," she shouted. "Let's go to the
beach."

Kellie drove. The beach was two hours away, and as we
wound through miles and miles of clear-cut forests, I leaned

into her and clutched her arm. It was hard for me to leave an inch of space between us. Whenever I was near her, my body wanted to lean in.

"I ordered some babies for us," she joked. "They should be arriving any day now."

I liked the joke. I wanted her to want that. I treated it as some kind of promise, though in the months that followed she didn't speak again of babies.

In bed that morning in our cabin, after Kellie asked if I was sure, she sat up in bed, laced her fingers together and stretched her arms as far as they would go. I watched as her shoulder blades stretched and then returned to their place. "Coffee?" she asked. As she rose, she left behind a heap of rumpled sheets.

Up until now, I had held these truths, one in each hand: I wanted a child. I wanted to be with Kellie. I had made no room for a conflicting truth: Kellie had never agreed to have children.

2
ACCIDENTALLY
ON PURPOSE

Sometimes straight people have exhaustive discussions about whether or not they want to become parents. Sometimes they take months or even years to lay plans and reconsider, to toss around ideas about how to pay for daycare, where the crib should go, and who will change the diapers.

Sometimes they do this. Often they don't. Often, for better for worse, straight couples just go ahead and have kids. Sometimes conception happens by accident: a condom breaks, an IUD fails. Sometimes conception happens kind-of-on-purpose, as in, let's try just this once and see what happens. Sometimes bodies, in the heat of a moment, make a choice while the prefrontal cortex, lulled by arousal, is too tranquil to protest.

When we talk about planned and unplanned pregnancies, we act like there's a distinct line that divides the two. On one side are the babies who arrived in this world through a clear act of intention. On the other side are the unexpected babies. But this is not the case. Line the babies up, and you have a spectrum, a whole range between planned and unexpected, with most of them sitting somewhere in the middle.

One recent study suggested that women applied birth control less consistently when they were sleeping with men who had "preferred mating characteristics."[4] The more attractive the man was, the more intelligent, the more family-oriented, the less likely the woman was to consistently use or insist on birth control. Instead, she took her chances, presumably deciding—consciously or not—that a baby might be a favorable outcome.

Another study showed that women who wanted to have children eventually were far less likely to choose long-acting reversible contraceptives such as IUDs and implants.[5] In other words, the woman who says she wants a child in three years is not so likely to choose a form of birth control that will support this plan with near certainty. In one sense, this isn't rational. If you know you want a child in three years, why not make sure that you won't get pregnant early? In another sense, these decisions perfectly follow the heart's wily logic: sometimes we want to leave a little room in life for our dreams to surprise us. We might not actually want total control of our life's course.

According to a Pew Research Poll, nearly half of all parents, when asked why they decided to have children, answered, "There wasn't a reason; it just happened."[6]

For most lesbian couples, a baby can't "just happen." Nearly all of the babies born to lesbian parents sit at the *planned* end of the baby lineup. I say *nearly* because there are sapphic couples where one partner is trans and has sperm to offer or couples that are nonmonogamous where one or both partners sleep with men on occasion. And I'm sure that somewhere out there, there are lesbian couples with willing male friends who got pregnant on a whim, a lark at the end of joyful or raucous evening. But, for the most part, lesbians as a group must approach parenthood with intention and caution.

For many, this is not only because of the biological hurdle but because we don't have a clear vision of queer parenthood. I grew up knowing that, in theory, lesbians could become parents, but I had never known a family with two moms. I had never seen one on TV or read about one in a book. Decades after fifth grade, via the magic of social media, I would learn that Helen—my teacher who was rumored to be a "lezzie"—had been planning a family during the time I was her student. In the years that followed, she conceived with donor sperm and bore one child. Her partner later bore another. But as a child and young adult, I didn't know this. Helen's sexuality had been a whispered secret, and I could barely imagine her with a partner, never mind a baby. So often that's how queerness operates: we are told it exists, but the evidence is withheld. Queer families may be everywhere, but they are often unseen.

Kellie, who had always (in her adult life) been part of a vast queer community, had a couple of queer friends who were raising children as single mothers, but she knew no queer couples who were raising kids together. The role of adoptive mom who would parent side by side with a gestational mom was undefined and frightening to her, a role that came with no guarantees. Would she love her child automatically? Would her lack of biological connection be meaningful and obvious? Would it pain her? Kellie barely spoke of these fears. Instead, our discussion was coded. When she said, "I hope our babies look like you," I took it to mean: "I hope they don't look like a stranger." I picked up her fear and carried it. We had never heard anyone speak of such things.

Kellie had her own private feelings to consider and then also the reaction of the world at large. When straight couples decide to become parents, they must worry about money and space and careers and how they will navigate gender roles. Queer people, like those in other marginalized groups, must consider all of these same things and more: We don't know how our children will be treated or who might try to take them from us. We don't know how our kids will feel growing up being asked, "Where's your dad?" or "Why do you have two moms?"

In the years after I married Kellie, I felt a tinge of jealousy any time a straight woman I knew revealed a pregnancy that was both welcome and unexpected. "It just kind of happened," an acquaintance might say, one hand on the round of her belly. I wished that a pregnancy could just kind of happen to me, that I wouldn't have the pressure of thinking it all the way through and timing it perfectly. I suspected that, because I was a lesbian and because it was obvious that any baby I made was on purpose, people might assess my life choices with more scrutiny.

Some months before my wedding, when my relationship to Kellie was new and I couldn't contain my bliss, I confessed to my mother that I was tempted to have a baby right away. We were at an outdoor cafe when I said it. I was drinking coffee as my mother finished her lunch, and the caffeine had brought forth my longing and made me want to share. "Sometimes I feel so ready," I said, and my mother straightened in her chair.

She looked at me, wide-eyed and upright, a salad leaf poised on her fork. "I don't know why you'd want to do that," she said. Her tone was cold.

In that moment I saw myself through her eyes. I was only twenty-three. I had no career prospects. In college, I had studied French and literature, and now I was making rent each month by working at the bakery and teaching in an after-school French program. I wasn't on the fast track to anything. The things that worried my mother were the same things that made me want a child right away. I didn't know exactly what I wanted from life, but I knew that I wanted to be a parent. What if I led with the thing I wanted? What if I treated parenthood not as the end point of the journey to adulthood, but the beginning?

But I sensed clearly that if I had a baby too soon, I would disappoint my mother, and my mother was a stand-in for the world. Her judgment was the world's judgment. Her approval was the world's approval. Her face that day, blanched and horri-fied, would follow me. It would inform a game that I began to play with my body, a game of longing for a child while training myself to wait for a sensible moment—a moment that I could tell my mom that I was pregnant and watch her fill with joy, not dread.

While I waited, I tried to build a home in other ways.

I moved in with Kellie, and within six months we had adopted two dogs together—first a fat corgi with giant ears named Henri and then a rangy heeler mix named Winston. They slept on dog beds right outside our bedroom door, and when I woke at night, I listened for their snores and sighs. They both shed year-round. Kellie, who had once been able to keep her house immaculate, now compulsively swept the piles of white fur that accumulated daily.

Shortly after the dogs and I had settled in, I received a check in the mail from my father for $10,000. His family had owned a wheat farm in Walla Walla for generations. When I was a child, we flew across the country to visit Walla Walla, and we'd driven along the road named after my great-grandfather. I had seen the house along the creek where my father had spent his childhood summers and the rainbow over the barn door that my grandfa-ther had painted many decades ago. But now the family farm had been sold—hence the check.

I was happy for the money but sad for the loss, and Kellie understood. There was a road in Olympia named after her own family, and on that road she could point out houses that had once belonged to great-aunts and great-uncles. There had once been nothing between those houses but farmland. Now those homes were owned by strangers, and much of the farmland had been filled in with new dwellings.

And so we agreed that we would buy land together, that we would build our own family legacy. We hadn't yet agreed on children, but for some unspoken reason, it felt right to both of us to think this way, to want to set aside something that we could make ours now and hand off to future loved ones. Our future kin already existed as figments in the far reaches of our imaginations.

Kellie scoured the classifieds for land for sale, and every weekend we loaded our dogs in the back of Kellie's truck and drove over mountains until we reached faraway counties where the sky was clear and land was cheap. We looked at parcels in Naches, Tri-Cities, Cle Elum, Dayton, and Sunnyside. We drove east enough times to fall in love with the Old Thorp Highway, a stretch of road between Horlick and Ellensburg that ran along the Yakima River through groves of aspens and cottonwoods. In the summer, when the air was warm and dry, the cottonwoods gave off a particular smell—a smell that somehow captured the sticky softness of the seeds and the smooth silver of the bark. We got used to pitching tents and half sleeping through the night at whatever campground we found, waking to a tent full of dog breath.

Toward the end of summer, we found ourselves looking over a green valley on a plot of land that was surrounded by ponderosa forests. The patch of land itself was a steep hillside of yellow grass, jagged outcrops, and wild currant shrubs. A stand of aspens—the cottonwood's cousin—grew along the south side of the property. A good third of them were dead and covered with woodpecker holes. The rest had silver-dollar leaves that shimmered at the slightest breeze.

It was in the most inconvenient location we'd visited so far: three hundred miles and two mountain passes from Olympia, five hours of driving to a small town called Tonasket, another half an hour up SR 20, and then six miles up a rutted dirt road. But it was cheap, and it felt right, and so we bought it.

Across the valley, on the opposite hill, our neighbor was a former airplane mechanic who kept horses now and lived with his mother. He went by the names Dave and Fred interchangeably. Dave-Fred made his living now by building cabins for the city folk who wanted to see the wilderness on weekends. His biceps were nearly as large as his head, and he carried a pistol in a holster at his waist. Kellie and I paid him to frame a small cabin; we planned do the finish work ourselves.

In the evenings, as we watched the sun sink behind the hills, we heard mother cows low for their young. In the mornings, we woke to the sounds of hooves and munching grass; Dave-Fred had begun to let his horses roam free, and they became fond of our hillside. On the first weekend they showed up, Kellie drove the twenty-six miles to town to buy a giant silver trough for them. She hauled it in the back of her truck and placed it twenty feet from where we showered. Two of the more assertive horses, Stinky and Bob, wouldn't wait for it to fill. They drank directly from the hose as Kellie patted their muzzles. I laughed from the safety of the porch.

It took us three years to finish our cabin. We put up siding, installed floors, built a deck, and stained all the wood, inside and out. Kellie had spent her life using power tools. I had never touched them, but now I found a certain comfort in kneeling on the floor, pressing the nail gun to the boards over and over, and hearing the satisfying *thwap* each time a nail connected plank to subfloor. We were making something permanent and ours. Some evenings, as we sat on the front porch and watched the clouds light up and turn pink, I imagined a completed cabin and a child throwing sticks across the grass for the dogs.

I felt certain that if Kellie could simply agree to parenthood via her body and not her mind, if we could simply slip beneath the sheets one day and be careless, then we might have avoided any conflict. A child might have simply "just happened." I wished that such a life change might come to me suddenly, easily, without me even having to ask. But I did have to ask. I had to ask a lot and keep asking.

3
WAYS OF SAYING YES

It's a Saturday morning. Kellie's reading in bed. The window is cracked, and the cool morning air comes rolling in. It's sunny, or it's raining, or it's gray and dry outside. I carry two cups of coffee, one in each hand, steady, my eyes trained on the rims. Kellie takes her cup from me and slurps the first sip. I taste my own and place it on the bedside table. I settle into bed. I grab whatever book I'm reading—*Like Life*, or *Lost in the City*, or *Charity*—but I don't open it. "So," I begin.

"What?" Kellie asks. She knows what's coming.

"Any thoughts?"

She sighs. She puts down her book. "All the same ones," she says.

"No new ones?"

"Are we having this conversation again?" she asks.

"Yes," I say. I rest my own book on top of my legs. I'm trying to pull from Kellie the answer I need. I treat it like that magic trick where the magician pulls a long rope made of tied-together kerchiefs from his mouth. If I keep pulling, eventually I will get to the end.

"I will probably never be sure," she says.

"I know that," I say. "I don't need you to be at one hundred percent."

"But I have misgivings," she reminds me.

"What now?" I ask. I want her to enumerate her objections so I can bury them. I want to dig a tiny grave for each one.

"We're destroying our planet," Kellie says. We've discussed this before, and in the abstract I see her point—that we are a planet exploding with human bodies, bodies that consume and make waste, bodies that pollute the oceans and the rivers. Like vermin, we multiply and overtake. I see this, but it doesn't change what I want.

"So you just want to give up?" I say. "Like we should all just stop having kids?"

"I don't know," she says.

"That seems hopeless."

"I just don't like people that much. I like animals."

I think back to the first time I noticed Kellie, her dog Rusty in the passenger's seat, happy and panting. I think about the day we had to put Rusty down and how Kellie left the exam room with her hand shielding her eyes. I think about the time we were visiting friends on their ranch and as I looked out their window one morning I saw Kellie emerge with something tucked beneath her coat. When she opened it, an owl flew out. It had been trapped in the barn, she explained to me later. She had scooped it up and set it free, just like that. I'm not sure that Kellie's deep connection to the animal world is evidence that she'd be a bad parent. It's true that kids are people, but it's true that they're animals too.

"You would probably like your own kid. You might like your kid more than any dog you've ever had."

"What if I don't?"

If I look closely enough, I can see the genuine fear in her eyes. When she blinks, she lets her eyelids rest for an extra moment.

"I'm willing to take that risk," I say.

I lean to my side and stare out the window for a minute. I entertain a fantasy, one where Kellie and I have broken up and I've gone on to have a child with someone else. In this dream I'm in Kellie's front yard—I've stopped by because I'm in the neighborhood. I have a two-year-old with big eyes and wild hair on my hip. The kid plays with the collar of my shirt while Kellie and I talk. It's sunny out. Kellie and I stand ten feet apart. The distance between us crackles. We can't quite meet each other's eyes. In my fantasy, Kellie is looking at my child and thinking, *I could have done that after all.* But it is too late.

"I just want it to be you," I tell her now. "I want that."

"What's wrong with us the way we are now?" she asks.

"Nothing's wrong," I say. "But not having a kid doesn't feel like a choice for me."

"So you'll leave me if I don't agree?"

"Is that the way you want to see it?" I ask.

This is the reel that ran in our bedroom every weekend, the same argument looped over and over, week after week after week. Each time we arrived at the same conclusion: I wanted a child. Kellie wasn't sure. We could take the discussion no further. Eventually we would give up on talking. I would try to read, but the words in my brain would jumble with the words on the printed page. I would leave the bed, eat breakfast, and join Kellie later in the yard.

In this way, we resumed our weekend. Outside, Kellie watered the garden beds while I picked raspberries and dropped them into a plastic tub. Occasionally, the spray from the hose would graze my ankle. When I finished collecting the raspberries, I held the tub below her face. She took a handful. The quiet between us was generous. We planned to be okay. We didn't know how we would get there, but somehow we would.

One Saturday night, after dark, we spread out on the couch to watch a movie. Kellie rested her head on the armrest and, though it wasn't comfortable, I nestled in behind her. As the opening credits rolled, I whispered in her ear. "I have an idea," I told her.

"About what?" she asked.

"The baby," I said.

"Okay," she said and waited.

"Let's say we have a baby and you don't love it right away. We can just dress it in a bunny suit."

Together we pictured a baby asleep in a crib, wearing a cottontail and floppy pink ears. I imagined us sharing the exact same image in both of our imaginations, as if I had telepathically transferred it from my mind to hers. "Look—a bunny," Kellie said.

"Exactly," I said. "That would work, wouldn't it?"

"That would probably work," she conceded.

I threaded my fingers through hers and tried to settle into watching the movie, but I was dreaming now, my mind's eye fixed on that sleeping baby dressed in white fleece, his back rising and falling with breath.

Sometimes I asked her, "You knew I wanted to have a child when you married me, didn't you?"

She said she'd figured we'd work it out one way or another.

Sometimes I said, "If we were straight, we'd just do it."

She said if we were straight we'd already have three kids by now.

Often Kellie ended the conversation by throwing up her hands. "We're doing this whether I want to or not, so fine."

"That's not a yes," I told her. "If you want to tell me you're scared but you're willing, that's one thing. But that's not what you're saying."

In a neighborhood park one day, I brought my complaints to an older friend named Nancy. We took turns throwing a ball for our dogs and watching them race and leap to catch it. The winner would deposit a slobbery ball at our feet, and both of them would sit, mouths open, tongues lolling out, their full attention focused on the object. Nancy liked to tease our dogs by poking at the ball with her foot and watching them flinch in anticipation.

Nancy wanted me to have a baby. She wanted Kellie to agree. On previous dog outings, she had spent time listing all of the straight couples she knew who had kids in spite of uncertainty. She told me about what good parents they were, about how she wished she'd had a child of her own, about how our independent lives don't always pan out the way we think they will. She said this as someone who had divorced at the age of forty-one, who had come out late in life, and who had spent the last seven years working on a dissertation that she feared she'd never finish. Though Nancy, with her cool eyes and cropped hair, looked like a person you wouldn't want to mess with, she spoke in a voice so gentle and cooing, I always wanted to lean in.

On this day, I told Nancy about Kellie's most recent stance of exasperation, of saying yes when she clearly didn't mean it, and then I described my response. "I told her that I didn't need her to be sure, but I needed her to be willing."

My dog had caught the last pitch and he was now bounding toward us, victorious.

"Or she could say *no*," Nancy pointed out. "I notice you left out that option."

I picked up the slobbery ball and held it for a moment. I looked at it. There was a rope of dog saliva on one side, some grit where the ball had hit the ground. I looked at Nancy, trying to take in what she had just said. It was something I had never accounted for: a clean no. Though I had imagined that moment of reckoning on the lawn, the one where Kellie met the child that might have been hers, I had never filled in the rest of that imagined future, an actual life without Kellie. I had never acknowledged, not fully, that Kellie had a right to walk away. I didn't want that to be true. In the years we'd been keeping house together, driving to and from the cabin, I had always imagined a child arriving at some point. I thought Kellie did too. Some part of me had treated these discussions like a mere formality, a hoop we had to jump through to arrive at our destined life.

I had no words for Nancy. I just looked at her blankly and threw the ball for the dogs as worry continued to swell in my chest.

Sometimes Kellie imagined scenarios that would please her. "If my brother would help us, I'd do it in a heartbeat," she offered. Or: "If I knew for sure we'd have a girl, I'd be okay."

Still, she got stuck on all the outcomes we couldn't control. She told me about Serena, a challenging six-year-old who used to live in the neighborhood. Serena's mother came over with unwashed hair and dark circles under her eyes. At night, she had to lock Serena in her bedroom to keep her from destroying the house. In Kellie's backyard one day, Serena kicked Kellie's dog so hard she yowled in pain and hid beneath the porch for hours.

I had no answer for this concern except that I was willing to take all of the risks. I couldn't promise Kellie that our child would be kind and bright and easy to love. It was true that our child might be a Serena—a small person who was worthy of love but who would also demand everything you had: all of your time, all of your money, and all of your patience, and when those things dried up, she would still demand more. I couldn't promise her otherwise, but I could state my belief, over and over, that the odds were in our favor, that our child might be just as likely to hold Kellie's face in between her small hands as she would be to kick our dogs.

"I'll have to work this job forever," was another one of Kellie's objections. She worked Monday through Friday from 7:00 a.m. to 3:30 p.m. as a maintenance electrician. That extra half hour was tacked on to the end of her day to compensate for the half-hour lunch break she didn't want to take. "Can't you just skip it and get off at three?" I'd asked her once. "No," she had said. "I asked." She worked in the heat and the cold and the rain, but it wasn't so much the hours she minded or the weather. What she minded was not having enough to do. There were plenty of days when there was little to maintain, when she drove around looking for light bulbs to change or sat at a desk and updated work orders. She minded that she gave so much of her life to a place that paid her well but didn't seem to need her the way she wanted to be needed. She dreamed of making some radical change—of making a living restoring houses or caretaking a ranch in some far-off wilderness—but those options seemed blurry and out of reach in our current situation. We had no nest egg or business plan, just a home equity loan we'd maxed out to build the cabin. Kellie clung to security more than she wanted to, and having a child in the picture would only amplify that.

"You can quit," I told her.

"How would that work?" she asked me.

I didn't have an answer. I had just spent two years in graduate school pursuing a degree in creative writing. Mostly I had done it for love, but I had hoped it might magically lead to a practical career. While I was there, I'd been paid to teach first-year students, but now that the program was over, I was back to working at the bakery for eight dollars an hour plus tips. Clearly I wasn't the breadwinner.

In the end, it was a small purchase that settled the matter, an impulse buy of sorts.

It was September by then and, almost miraculously, I'd been

offered a job teaching English at a community college less than a week before the school year started. Every day now, I did my best impersonation of an organized professional. I wore collared shirts, stood in front of twenty-eight students, and talked about things like thesis statements and sentence fragments. One afternoon I came home from work to an empty house. From the kitchen window, I could see Kellie outside, raking the debris that had fallen from the cedar tree in our backyard.

I set a pot of water to boil for dinner, and then I went to the bedroom to change out of my work clothes. That's where I saw what she had left for me: a bunny suit, white and fluffy with pink ears, laid out in the middle of the bed.

"What's this?" I asked Kellie once she came inside. I had moved the bunny suit to the kitchen, where I draped it over the back of a chair. The hood of the suit framed a shadow where a face would go, and the ears pointed down to the floor. I wanted to know what Kellie would say. Did she have a yes for me, finally?

"I just saw it in the window of that consignment shop in town," she said.

"Oh," I said. I moved over to the stove to check the water. Small bubbles rose to the surface, and steam gathered, but it was still some moments away from reaching a true boil.

"I thought we might need it someday," she said.

4
BODY LORE

I assumed I had a fertile body, that the desire I felt to bear a child was a chemical that traveled through my bloodstream, that it informed my eggs, my ovaries, my uterus. I assumed that in those dark places, everything was ripening, opening, preparing. I assumed that the moment semen entered my body, I would be instantly, irrevocably pregnant. I assumed that negotiations with Kellie would be the only obstacle between me and my future child.

Over the course of my childhood, my mother had convinced me that I came from a line of exceptionally fertile women. The story of my own conception goes like this: My parents were not married. They had recently reunited after a breakup. My mother, ever careful, was faithfully using birth control. She got pregnant anyways. A determined sperm swam past a diaphragm and reached a welcoming egg. As I grew inside my mother's womb, my parents discussed whether or not they would keep me. My father wasn't certain, but my mother was. They settled on yes and decided to marry. As a fetus, I gave my mother eight weeks of morning sickness but never a reason to worry she might lose me.

There were other family stories. My grandmother conceived my mother on her wedding night and then conceived an unplanned third child when she was in her midthirties. My half sister, my father's child from an earlier marriage, conceived her son after one attempt at the age of thirty-six.

All around me, people spoke of fertility as if it were a virtue. "If I so much as look at a dick, I get pregnant," a friend bragged to me once. "I bet you'd get pregnant in a heartbeat," is the sort of compliment I've overheard straight men bestow on their girlfriends, thus conflating their beauty, desire, or vibrancy with their potential fertility.

When the female body is commodified, its ability to produce more bodies becomes an essential part of its value. Women become more receptacle than human. Under patriarchy, a woman's body is a vessel for men's pleasure and a vessel for growing progeny—and those are its primary uses. That a woman's body has value simply for the pleasure and function it offers its owner has not been so widely considered or acknowledged. Women who can't bear children have historically been referred to as barren, conjuring images of depleted farmland—something that once had value made valueless.

Culturally, we tend to conflate three disparate things: sexual desire, the impulse to nurture, and the ability to conceive and bear a child. We act as if a woman's longing is proportionate to her fertility. I longed deeply, and therefore I was fertile—or so my logic went.

It never occurred to me that for every story I heard about easy conceptions, there was an equivalent story—often whispered or untold—of failed attempts, of interventions, of miscarriages, and of giving up. I didn't think about those who struggled to conceive and how they were just as alive with desire as those who made babies without trying. If I had asked around, I might have learned that my great-grandmother wed to legitimize a pregnancy she would later lose. I might have learned about the aunt who tried for years to conceive and then finally gave up. Or, if I had reflected for even a moment, I would have remembered a dear aunt who had lost three consecutive pregnancies while I was growing up. The first one ended early, but the second two losses had come in the middle of the second trimester. She had named the children she would never raise and buried their remains beneath a tree in her backyard. I knew about her losses not because she spoke of them openly, but because each time she miscarried, she called my mother. I came to recognize the sound of her crying voice, muffled through the receiver.

But while my aunt's misfortunes may have touched me, they didn't prompt me to reconsider my assumptions about fertility. As a child, this aunt had loved me as well as any grown-up in my life. She invited me for long weekend visits in her home where her cooking steamed up the windows, where houseplants thrived, and where her golden retriever lay happily on the sofa. If fertility were truly correlated to maternal instinct, she would have conceived instantly. But of course these two things aren't related. We know this—I knew it—but we carry on believing anyways. I had convinced myself that I was exceptionally fertile. I didn't let reality get in the way of my optimism.

II.

5
POSITIONS

Kellie and I had different positions on sperm.

My position was that it didn't matter. It was just an ingredient we needed, like sugar for a cake. I wanted it fast, and I wanted it easy—I wasn't too interested in the source. If, say, our local convenience store had carried the product, if they had a shelf in their freezer next to the Klondike Bars and Rocket Pops dedicated to tiny vials of processed semen, I would have happily purchased it there. I would have slid open the freezer door, reached in, and pulled out whatever sample lay on top of the stash. When I got to the counter, I might have added a Milky Way bar just to distract the clerk from my main purchase. I would have laid down my cash, wished them a nice day, and walked home with the vial tucked into the palm of my hand. Along the way I might have finally peeked at the label. 6840: Italian American donor with blue eyes and black hair. Five foot nine. *Cool,* I would have thought. 7954:

Salvadorian donor with brown eyes and wavy hair. Five foot seven. *Nice.*

In reality, because semen requires cryogenic storage, Don's EZ Mart didn't carry it. But ordering sperm from a catalog would only be slightly more complicated. We would just need a couple of hours, a catalog from a reputable sperm bank, a pencil to mark our top picks, and a credit card. I saw no reason to make it any harder than it needed to be.

For me, initially, treating sperm like a non-precious commodity felt strategic. Our donor wouldn't be our child's father, so why invest too much emotional energy in choosing him? Some part of me felt that if I cared too much about the source of our child's DNA, I'd be valuing nature over nurture and, in doing so, setting Kellie up to be a less important parent.

But Kellie's position on sperm was that it mattered a lot. We were choosing DNA that would stand in for her genetic material. Because she was in no rush to make a baby, efficiency wasn't a selling point. What she wanted was connection. Kellie hated the idea of choosing a donor from a catalog, of selecting a number rather than a human.

"Just be open to it," I pleaded. "Maybe you'll find a profile you like."

"What's a profile going to tell me?" she asked. "Who are these people? How do I know they're not just jerks off the street?"

"Because they're screened," I insisted. The moment I said it, I wondered what that meant. Did these men arrive at some brightly lit office and fill out a questionnaire in #2 pencil? Was their place of employment verified? Were they in it for the cash? I had wanted to believe that the process of sperm donation would attract men who were kind and bright, men for whom being paid to masturbate was just a minor perk compared to the joy of helping people make babies.

"I just don't like it," Kellie told me.

I didn't realize it at the time, but Kellie's mistrust of sperm banks was grounded in their complex and undeniably patriarchal history. Kellie understood intuitively that sperm banks are (in most cases) a business, not a community asset.

Kellie was convinced it would be better to find our own donor, someone we knew and respected, someone we found handsome and clever, who knew how to use a jigsaw, who could fix a leaking gasket and frame a window, but also someone who read books and didn't turn into an asshole after a couple of beers. Also, he would need to have the right attitude—open to the idea of sharing his sperm, and possibly interested in knowing the resulting kid, but not too interested. He could become a friend to our future child, or maybe even an uncle, but not an actual father. He could drink coffee with us on Saturday mornings, he could call the kid *buddy* and tousle his hair, but after an hour or so, we'd want him to check the time and say, *I'd better get going.* He would have to be mature enough and introspective enough to commit to that distance, to not change his mind when the baby was born and decide he wanted custody.

"Can't you see what a long shot that is?" I asked Kellie one morning. The discussion had started in the bedroom, and when the tension rose, we had moved to the kitchen, where I now sat across from her. There was nothing between us but a stretch of table. "Look," she said, reaching for my hand. Her grip was firm; it calmed me. "I don't really think those donors are assholes. I just want our kid to be a little like me. And I want to be able to look our donor in the eye and know that he's a good person."

I nodded. I didn't want to deny her that. "We can try to find someone," I told her.

I was twenty-nine already. I didn't feel old, but I was feeling less young, and I had just agreed to wander down what I suspected was a dead-end road.

6

THE SHORT LIST

Kellie and I agreed on a list of possible donors.

Our top choice was a no-brainer. Kellie's brother Ron lived just on the other side of town with a wife and two kids. He owned a contracting business, worked out at the gym every morning, and drove a new white truck that he kept pristine. I could describe him as a man's man, but there was also a tenderness to him. When he lifted his own sons to greet them, he held them for a long moment before letting them go. In a lot of ways, Ron was like Kellie, who would have also been a man's man if she'd been a man at all.

Over the years, we had brought the idea up with him, but never in earnest. One Christmas Eve, years earlier, we found ourselves with Ron and his wife in their kitchen. As we put away food, scraped plates, and stacked dishes, Ron's wife prodded us. "What about kids?" she asked. "We want nieces and nephews."

Kellie didn't hold back. "Yeah, we might have kids. You want to help us with that, Ronnie?"

Ron kept his attention on the dishes in the sink. Without looking up, he said, "You don't want that."

"No, actually, I do," was Kellie's answer. She took a plate from her brother's hand and loaded it into the dishwasher.

"Nah," he went on. "That would just be too weird. I don't want any more kids out there in the world."

"They wouldn't be yours, they'd be mine," Kellie said.

"Yeah," he concluded. "I just think it would be weird."

I knew, in a way, that Ron was right. The situation would not be un-weird. We were asking for his semen, which he would have to hand over to us every month until we conceived. That would be the short-term weird, finite and defined. But then there would also be the long-term weird, the family gatherings where everyone would know that Uncle Ron was, biologically speaking, not an uncle but a father. We might never speak of it, but how would our hearts feel? Would Ron feel a tug? If so, how strong? Would it be the kind of twinge you could ignore?

We knew it would be weird, but for us, the value so obviously outweighed the weirdness. For Ron, it so obviously didn't.

But that conversation had happened years ago, and the situation had been hypothetical. Now that it was real, Kellie and I agreed we'd give it an honest try. Kellie wrote a letter in pencil on lined notebook paper. The letter said, *I am afraid to become a parent, but I want to. If you could do this for me, I would be less afraid.* On a Friday morning, she drove by Ron's house on her way to work. He was already gone, and so she opened the door to his mailbox. Later in the day, the mail carrier would drive by and leave the usual pile of bills and coupons. In the evening, when Ron returned home, it would be the last thing he came to as he sorted through the stack: a plain, white envelope with his first name in his sister's writing. Maybe he read it alone at his kitchen table, an open beer at his side. Or maybe he read it with his kids tugging at his pants or climbing on his back.

The next morning, Ron knocked on our door. I hovered behind Kellie as she answered. It was 10:00 a.m. and the sun shone brightly behind him, just beyond our front porch. Ron looked earnest and shaken, like he might burst open and fall apart if you touched him even gently. I didn't know how to act. "Oh, hey," I said, "How's it going?" I slipped into the kitchen, where I put the kettle on for coffee. I wasn't sure that anyone would drink it, but I needed an excuse to fumble around, to reach above me for the filters, to pour the beans and run the grinder so that, for a few moments at least, I could drown out their conversation and collect myself instead. As I poured hot water over the grounds I prayed: *Say yes, say yes, say yes.* I pictured babies that looked like Kellie, kids with olive skin and striking eyes who liked the sun and the dirt. I pictured Kellie and me holding a baby between us, knowing that when we said "our baby," the "our" was unconditional, that our baby's blood carried ties not just to my own ancestors, but hers as well.

I would never hear Ron's thoughts that day.

Moments after I finished making coffee, we were interrupted by some unexpected guests. Geri and Richard—Kellie's mother and stepfather—pulled into our driveway. They emerged from the car, smiling. They were in the neighborhood and thought they'd stop by. It was a bizarre coincidence. They lived in a waterfront home forty minutes away, and so it wasn't that we never saw them, but they rarely came to us. Instead, we often made the drive to visit them. When we came over, Geri—always in styled platinum hair and red lipstick—put on an apron and baked. In her kitchen she recounted to Kellie all the recent happenings of family members and neighbors. Geri had a sailor's mouth. "Al's boat went tits up last week," she might report, or, "For crap's sake, I wish Mitzi's husband would get his act together." While she talked, I sat awkwardly on the edge of her white sofa, trying to blend in. I was never sure what Kellie's family thought of me. They were a clan who spoke loud enough to be heard, who easily started conversations with strangers, who didn't overthink every last social interaction. They never seemed to judge me, but I worried that my shyness didn't make sense to them. And so today, as I stepped off the porch to greet them, I tried to be easy.

"Look who's here!" Geri said after spotting her son. She offered me a quick hug and then seemed to read my face. "Did we interrupt something?" she asked us.

"No," Ron answered.

Inside, I placed a cup of coffee in everyone's hand and hoped that Ron might outlast Geri and Richard, that he might stick around long enough that we'd get down to the conversation we'd already spent some minutes avoiding. But I should have known better. When Ron finished his coffee, he set his cup down on the table and rose. "Mom," he said, before offering her the first parting hug. "Richard," he said, and then, "Jenn," and then, "Kellie," each of us named before his departure. He didn't need to explain himself. He was there, and then he was gone. We never spoke of it again.

We explored other possibilities. There was Alex, a craftsman Kellie had worked with on a remodeling project. He was goofy but handsome, with jet-black hair, big hands, and a remarkably deep voice. It had been a few years since we'd seen him, but he was close with some friends we kept up with, Susan and Mark. We schemed with them one afternoon as we sat on stools in their kitchen. They would run the scenario by him but wouldn't mention us by name, they promised.

Two weeks later, they reported their news to us, both of them laughing and hopeful. Mark told us about the conversation they'd had just a few days earlier. "So, how would you feel if you knew a lesbian couple who wanted a baby..." they'd begun.

Alex didn't wait for them to finish. "Kellie and Jenn are having a baby?" he asked.

We all laughed over this. It seemed like a good sign that he remembered us, even if his response suggested we were the only lesbians he'd ever known.

Mark continued his report. Apparently Alex had taken a moment to consider it. Then he nodded and concluded, "So that's cool. I guess that means I'd get to sleep with Jenn."

"I don't think it works that way," Susan had told him.

Kellie and I laughed. I hoped that no one noticed I was blushing or that for a full minute, I wasn't sure where to look. I focused on one leg of the coffee table while Kellie kept the conversation going. *I'd get to sleep with Jenn.* It was kind of sweet, maybe, or flattering, or funny. It was hard to know how Alex had meant it. Was he kidding, or did he genuinely assume that was what we had in mind? I pictured a bed that wasn't mine. I imagined myself in it: lying on my side, naked and waiting for a man I barely knew. I thought about what it would mean to make a child that way, by sleeping with a person outside of my marriage. I knew there were people in the world who did that, people who invited a donor into their bedroom. I wondered what that would mean for the partner, the person who was bound to love and raise this child in spite of the fact that it would not grow inside of them, nor would it share any of their DNA. To ask them to bear witness as an outsider penetrated their wife, or to ask them to be gone—to go for a walk while the other two filled the bedroom with human sounds and smells— that struck me as hopelessly lonely.

I knew that we could easily explain the process of sperm donation to Alex, that perhaps Susan had already set him straight, and yet I couldn't let it go. It mattered to me that he'd said what he said, that sex had entered the conversation. In my mind, our ideal donor was a man who intuitively knew to avoid that. It was true that, no matter what, sex was a part of this equation. I understood that our donor, anonymous or known, would need to ejaculate. He might do this in a bathroom with magazines or grab a cup and reach for the bottle of lotion by his bedside. Sometime later, I would lie naked in my own bed and receive this product via a needleless syringe. Some of the books I had read suggested I should aim to have an orgasm too, that doing so would open my cervical os—the tiny portal to my reproductive organs—and usher the sperm toward my egg. To make a baby this way was still a sexual act, even if there were miles between the actors. It was precisely because of this that I could only pretend to be fine with Alex's joke. I needed that aspect of the transaction—its connection to body and sex—to remain implicit, unspoken.

I wondered if I was overreacting. Maybe Kellie wouldn't care. Maybe I could get past it. On the car ride home, Kellie drove. Once we hit the freeway, I settled in the passenger's seat; I took off my shoes and pulled one knee up toward my chest. "So what do you think?" I asked.

"About Alex?"

"Yeah," I said. "I'm sure he was kidding."

"Maybe," Kellie said. She paused for a moment. "But he meant it." She looked steadily ahead. "He's out."

There was Kellie's coworker, whom she worked alongside most days. He had two daughters, blond girls aged four and one with big brown eyes and pigtails. "I'd be your donor," he offered one morning as they drove. "I've always wanted my kids to have a bunch of siblings," he went on. "It would be cool if you guys had a boy."

"I don't think he gets it," I told Kellie that night. "They wouldn't be his kids."

"He knows that," she said.

"Except he kind of doesn't," I shot back.

Kellie sighed.

There was my brother, Nick, who we asked as a kind of backup plan. As far as we knew, Kellie could get pregnant too. Pregnancy was never an experience she'd wanted or imagined for herself, but when we talked about the possibility of her carrying a child, she didn't rule it out. Her willingness surprised me, but the discussion always felt purely hypothetical. Besides her lack of interest, Kellie was approaching forty. Women her age got pregnant every day—we knew this—but both logically and intuitively, I was the real shoo-in candidate for gestation.

Nick had been a part my life with Kellie from early on. As a teenager fresh out of high school, he'd moved across the coast and lived with us briefly. It grounded me to have my little brother around. He wasn't little anymore—he was six foot six and had a habit of leaving his size 16 sneakers over our heater vent to dry out. We'd come home and wonder briefly why our house smelled like a locker room, and then we'd find the shoes underneath the kitchen table, the heater spreading their hot stink throughout the house. But in spite of his height and his stinky shoes, my brother didn't take up too much space. Mostly he slept late and read books on the couch and rode his bike to town and back. He bought vegetables and ate lots of chips and salsa. Having him around made my world feel a little bigger and more connected to love.

He didn't stay forever, though. He returned to the East Coast, where he found friends and work. Now he was planning a two-year return to Olympia so he could finish college and study organic farming.

I asked Nick at the tail end of a long-distance phone call. "I hope this isn't too weird," I began, "and we probably wouldn't even go this route, but would you ever consider being our donor? You know, like, if Kellie were going to carry." The words came out easily. Of all of the people we asked, Nick was the person I trusted most. I wasn't sure he'd say yes, but I knew that he'd be thoughtful and kind.

He paused for just a moment. "I'd have to think about it," he said.

The next time we spoke, he brought it up unprompted. "I thought about it," he said. "I'd do that."

I felt gratitude at his willingness, but it felt more like a blessing from an alternate universe than an actual possibility. The scenario we were discussing was the mirror image of what we thought we wanted most of all. Instead of me carrying a baby who was genetically tied to Kellie's family, Kellie would carry a baby that was genetically tied to mine. But it mattered that the mirror image was backwards. It mattered that Kellie would be forty in a few months, and it mattered that she preferred to not be pregnant.

There was Adam, an acquaintance we saw occasionally at parties. He and Kellie often attracted attention by unintentionally wearing matching outfits—Carhartt pants with a faded T-shirt and flip-flops in the summer or cable sweaters and knitted caps in the winter. At one of these parties, he had jokingly volunteered to be our eventual donor.

"Sign me up!" he had said. "I'd love to have kids I'm not responsible for."

"Careful," Kellie warned. "We'll remember you said that."

"No, I mean it," he said. "I'd be into it. I'd just drop off a bag of groceries once in a while, wave at your kids, and drive off."

Kellie and I talked about it afterward. We did not object to free groceries. We filed the information away for future use.

At the same friend's house some months later, Adam found us outside at a picnic table, sharing pie off a paper plate. He sidled over, set down his beer, and sat directly across from us. "You are just the woman I've been looking for," he told Kellie.

"Why's that?" Kellie asked.

"I need a wireman," he said. "I just bought an old house and the kitchen's all fucked up."

"I can help you," Kellie said. These were four words I heard her utter multiple times a week. Though Kellie often complained at the way her weekends filled up with side jobs that paid little or nothing, we both knew she loved being asked. Adam and Kellie spent the next minutes going over the details of the project, which gave me a chance to eat all of the pie, watch the sky turn from dusk to dark, and wonder when and how we might go about broaching the topic of sperm.

"So what's new with you two?" Adam's voice startled me from my thoughts.

"Not much," I said. I traced the edge of the plate with my index finger.

"That's not really true," Kellie cut in. "We're getting ready to have a baby soon."

Adam looked at me. "You're pregnant?" he asked.

"No," I said, shaking my head emphatically.

"No," Kellie clarified. "What I mean is that we're looking for a donor."

I looked up from my plate, my heart pounding and hopeful. I

loved Kellie in that moment for just going for it. But Adam's eyes darted back and forth between us. He was cornered. "Wow, that's got to be hard to find," he said. "I know I could never do that."

My stomach spun around a twinge of shame. I poked at the remaining crumbs of piecrust with a fork, hoping to disguise my embarrassment.

———————

As we explored these possibilities, I tried to put the time to use by learning about my body. I bought books about fertility. I learned simple things, things it seemed I should have always known. I learned that the fluids my underwear caught between periods had their own pattern and significance. Once my bleeding had tapered off, the books told me, I'd likely be dry for nearly a week. Gradually, I might notice an occasional milky-white fluid. A sudden gush of thin, watery mucus was a sign that my hormones were shifting, that my follicles were preparing an egg. I learned that slippery mucus—the kind that had once seemed suspect, random, and slightly disgusting—was actually something of a magical fluid, designed to feed sperm and guide it toward the waiting egg. I consulted at least four books, and each one gave it a different name: fertile mucus, egg-white mucus, slippery mucus—but my favorite term was *spin*, which came from the German term *spinnbarkeit*, but which also called to mind a spider, spinning her web and drawing in the creatures she needed for sustenance.

Weeks before I read the books, I might have felt privately embarrassed upon finding spin between my legs. Sometimes it appeared in the morning, and I'd wipe it away only to have more of it appear. It was unruly stuff that seemed to want to stick to my thigh or gather in my pubic hair. But now that I knew what it was, I felt a certain pride in it, my spin. I noted it lovingly on my calendar, and wondered why, in all the years I'd been alive and menstruating, I had never learned these simple facts about my own body.

But tracking my mucus was only one step in a complex system that became part of my daily routine. I ordered a special thermometer designed to reveal my body's rhythms.

This thermometer resembled the glass-and-mercury thermometers I used to stick under my tongue as a child, only this one was so fat and round it looked cartoonish. Every morning before I rose to use the bathroom or drank a sip of water, I reached for my bedside table and pulled it from its pink plastic case. I checked the time and sank back into my pillow. For five full minutes, I lay there with the thermometer's metal bulb pushing against the underside of my tongue. Once those minutes had passed, I held the thermometer up to the light, turning it until I could make out the line. I kept a chart, printed on office paper and folded in half, and a pen at my bedside. I meticulously noted that day's number and—this was the satisfying part—connected it to the day before. The idea was to capture my resting temperature over the course of the month. If

I did it correctly, and if my body abided, the chart would show an undeniable spike mid-cycle, a leap from, say, 98.3 to 98.8. The spike meant that my egg had burst.

In truth, the chart didn't tell me much that I couldn't have figured out easily by simply noting the dates of my periods and tracking my cervical mucus. If I wanted more precise information, there were little plastic kits I could order in the mail. They were like pregnancy tests in that I could pee into a cup and use a tiny dropper to saturate the test strip with urine. On these tests, the pink line signaled impending ovulation.

So there was no real reason for me to lie in bed for five minutes every morning with a metal bulb beneath my tongue. Sometimes I wondered why I continued to do it, day after day and month after month. Every time my period arrived, I tried to convince myself to skip a month, to let it go. Instead, I found myself at my computer, clicking *print*. Every month, my printer spat out a blank chart, warm and crisp. This chart would eventually reconfirm the thing I already knew: that I ovulated on day sixteen of each cycle.

I continued to chart my cycles with clinical precision because I found hope in the small act of connecting one dot to another, connecting each day to the next. It was as if, in that moment, I was drawing a line from my current life to a future life, making a map to another version of myself: a mother holding a child.

We had one possibility left on our list. Dee, a close friend of ours, had been working on a project with a contractor named Jesse. Dee felt personally invested in our success. Over the past few years, she'd become a member of our family. Dee lived with her dog in a tiny house on the other side of town and kept her life as simple as possible so she could follow her own whims and be useful to friends and family. Her friendship with Kellie allowed her to hit both of these targets at once. Kellie was constantly inventing large-scale projects that she couldn't do alone, and Dee was always game to help. Kellie could rarely recruit me to, for instance, help her deconstruct an abandoned three-seater outhouse she found in a blueberry field and then reconstruct it in our yard. I didn't have the strength, the know-how, or the interest, but Dee had all three. She showed up in pigtails and Carhartt overalls, trailed by her dog and eager to work.

Soon, Dee was often joining us on our weekend trips to work on the cabin, which meant that we spent countless hours together in Kellie's truck. Kellie drove, Dee's dog tolerated our dogs in the very back, amongst the tools, and Dee and I took turns riding shotgun while the other crammed into the back seat next to the cooler and the pile of duffel bags. To entertain ourselves, we often talked about the future. Kellie's truck was loud, and to hear each other, we all had to lean toward the center and shout.

"Forget about having a girl," Dee announced to us one day.

"You're going to wind up with two boys, and they're going to be so burly and wild that everyone will call them Smoke and Stump."

We were passing by a town called Liberty, an old mining town in the Wenatchee Mountains, and I pictured two teenage boys in flannel shirts, carrying hatchets and chopping wood. They would have fit right into the landscape. "Smoke and Stump," I said at the end of the daydream.

"Smoke and Stump," Kellie said.

"We're not actually naming our kids that," I announced, just to clarify.

"But I want to," Kellie countered.

Ever since then, Dee was woven into my vision of a future family, and she must have felt the same, since she made a point of keeping her eyes open for potential donors. The first friend she'd asked had already had a vasectomy, and now Jesse was her top nomination. Jesse was a contractor who was helping her build a studio in a friend's backyard, and they worked together nearly every day. He was a bachelor in his midthirties who dated a lot and didn't plan to settle down. Dee had already pitched our situation to him: Wouldn't it be cool for him to pass on his DNA but not have any strings attached? He agreed that it would be kind of cool and offered to come and meet with us, but first he was traveling to Hawaii.

Here's the funny thing: we were traveling to Hawaii too, with Dee, the very same week that he was. We could all have mai tais together, Dee suggested. No business, no talk about babies or sperm or STDs or contracts, just a few friends hanging out, getting to know each other. "Sure. Call me," was Jesse's reply.

Dee's idea for a meetup sounded perfect to me. I agreed to the "no business" stipulation in principle, but I held on to a fantasy. According to my past two charts, I was due to ovulate at some point on our trip, and I wondered if the stars might align for me. I knew I couldn't expect this, but what if, upon meeting us, Jesse was ready to commit? What if I mentioned that I was ovulating and he suggested we just go for it? I imagined how the scenario might unfold naturally, with barely any awkwardness. I pictured us on some beachside bar just after sunset, tipsy on cocktails. I pictured Kellie making a run to a drugstore tucked away in one of those tourist villas. She'd return with a needleless syringe, and we'd send Jesse off to the bathroom with a rinsed-out mai tai cup. He'd emerge, grin sheepishly, and hand Kellie the sample. Kellie and I would then retreat to our rented car while Dee and Jesse remained on the beach and watched the rest of the sky go dark.

In this fantasy, I'd return from Hawaii pregnant. I'd be a mother within the year. It would make such a good story, I half convinced myself that it was possible.

While we were in Hawaii, Dee left Jesse three voicemails, but he never called her back. Of course he didn't—he was busy surfing, hiking, mountain biking, and drinking beers with his friends. In real life, who would want to break away from a Hawaii vacation to socialize with a couple of lesbians who wanted your sperm?

And therein lay my quandary. From one angle I could see our request as sexy and adventurous. Who wouldn't want to offer up sperm to a lesbian couple? It would be a fun thing to mention at dinner parties or on a third date. From another angle, I could see our request as terrifying. We were like vampires, seeking the bodily fluid of an innocent human, offering nothing in return.

On our vacation, Kellie, Dee, and I stayed in a one-bedroom house in Hawaii, and the first morning I was there, I woke with the birds and drank my coffee alone on the terrace. It had poured all night and the bench was damp, but day had broken and the sky was clear. The sun, rising steadily, revealed a landscape I had only seen in photos and movies: banana trees and gardenias, birds of paradise and plumerias. I tried to take all of it in with each sip of my coffee—the sweet air, the chorus of birds, my solitude. Just inside the sliding doors, Kellie and Dee sat talking, reliving memories that predated my friendships with either of them. We had days ahead of us to talk and wander aimlessly, to read on the beach and swim in the warm water.

When I finally stood up, I felt a sudden trickle down my leg—the burst of watery fluid that signaled a shift in my cycle. Since I was wearing only my pajama pants, no underwear, there was nothing there to catch it. I felt embarrassed, even though I was alone.

That morning my chart had shown a slight dip in my

temperature. It was happening now, in my body. A tiny egg. I thought about how close I could be, just one yes away from a baby, just one microorganism. What was so special about sperm? It was everywhere, all the time, abandoned in condoms that had been tossed to the side of the road or soaked up in a tissue and discarded. It was a ubiquitous substance—why was it so hard to get some?

But this egg would complete its journey in the same way that every other egg before it had, from the very first one to burst forth when I was twelve years old. This egg would launch from my ovary all expectant and joyful, but there would be no sperm awaiting her. There would just be the follicles waving around like sea anemones. She'd hang out for a while, lonely and withering, until she was finally shunted away two weeks later, expelled in a tide of blood.

We finally met Jesse a full month later and sat with him in the afternoon sun. I brought him a beer, and he drank it. He asked us how the process worked and listened intently as I explained that he could either bank his semen at a fertility clinic, or, preferably, once or twice a month, when the timing was right, he could offer us a fresh sample in a jar.

"So, I'd have to be on call?" he asked, and Kellie tried to make him feel better about it, saying, "You could skip a month if you're busy."

"That's the part that would be hard for me." Jesse, not wanting to say no, told us that he'd take three weeks to think about it.

Three weeks passed, then four, and finally I called him and left a nervous voice mail. He called back and explained that he still needed more time.

Kellie continued to hope even though I'd already given up, and then finally, one day, Dee came over for a visit, and when we mentioned Jesse, she got quiet for a moment.

"Oh yeah," she said. "His girlfriend just got pregnant. She doesn't want him to do it."

"Oh," I said, and thought about how if I were a better person, I would probably feel something other than abject jealousy.

7
BINDERS FULL OF MEN

A manila envelope from the country's largest sperm bank arrived in my mailbox only three days after I called to request it. I tucked it under my arm and looked around me before returning to my front porch, as if one of my neighbors might catch me—as if there were something forbidden inside. I sat on the step and ran my finger through the envelope seam to unstick the glue. California Cryobank, the catalog said at the top, white letters on a royal blue background. This thing in my hands had come to me so easily. I had asked for it and, with the snap of a finger, there it was. I pulled out the rest. Below the company's name, there was a photograph. I'm not sure what I had expected—maybe a classic image of a baby growing in utero, maybe a mother looking into the eyes of her newborn child. But this photo featured two teenage boys wearing backpacks and smiling at the camera. They stood beneath a tree. It looked like an image I'd expect to see on a college catalog.

Kellie pulled into the driveway with her window rolled down. "Hey, lady," she said and stepped out of her truck.

"Hey," I said. My heart sped. I wanted to show her the catalog, but I didn't want to overwhelm her. I tried to hide my grin.

Kellie sat down next to me. "What's that?"

I handed it to her. "It's from that sperm bank in California," I said. "I called them."

Kellie didn't open it. She just held it in her lap.

I reached over and laid a finger on one of the faces on the cover. "Who is this supposed to be?" I asked her. "Are these the babies, all grown up?"

Kellie cocked her head and looked at me to make sure I was serious. "They're the donors," she said.

Shit. She was right. My excitement for the packet fizzled. These boys weren't what I had in mind. Whoever designed the cover must have hoped to convey that these were young men at the peak of their health, but all it highlighted for me was that many of these donors were too young to be making decisions of permanent consequence. They looked like boys, not men. Staring at the picture made me think of factory farming, of dairy cows hooked to milking machines, of chickens dropping eggs in chutes. Were these boys ready to commit to a lifetime of knowing there were children out there that they had helped create? I suspected that most of them just wanted the money for textbooks or beer.

Kellie lifted herself from the step to go inside. I propped the catalog on my knees. Moisture from my skin condensed on the back cover. I flipped through the pages aimlessly, my hope dim.

My position on sperm—my insistence that a sperm bank was our best and easiest option—was in part based on an assumption I had held since that day in my fifth-grade classroom when I learned about test-tube babies and concluded that modern medicine would help me conceive a child. I assumed that the fertility industry wanted to help me, that sperm banks had been designed with lesbians in mind.

I understood that straight couples and single women used sperm banks too, but I had always figured that lesbian couples would make a large share of their clientele, that sperm banks would welcome us, and that our needs would be built into the design of their operation.

I was wrong about this.

California Cryobank, one of the first commercial sperm banks, opened in 1977 with a very specific purpose: to offer men a way to store their own sperm for future use. This meant that, for instance, a man undergoing treatment for cancer could store vials of semen before starting chemo and radiation, and in doing so could hang on to the option of fathering children someday. Sperm storage was originally envisioned as a niche market for men, available mainly as a safeguard against future infertility.

Male sterility, the founders believed, had the potential to be psychologically "shattering"—devastating to a man's ego.[7]

Few were talking about male infertility as a widespread phenomenon. "Barren" was—and still is—a term applied only to women. Male infertility was seen as so profoundly emasculating that doctors barely mentioned it, even to each other. In the era predating the commercial sperm bank, if a couple had no luck conceiving a child, and if the microscope revealed that the husband's lack of sperm was at fault, doctors simply recruited one of their male students or staff to donate fresh semen. Sometimes the doctor himself was the secret donor. The arrangement was casual. In many cases, there was no documentation or paperwork. No STD testing. No legal safeguards. No washing, freezing, or quarantining. Just sperm from a source that would always be anonymous to the couple that received it. The prevailing attitude was: Just fix the problem. The less said, the better. This approach allowed the husband and wife to carry on as if they'd conceived the child unassisted. Many couples never spoke of the procedure again and never told their children.

It's worth noting that both this hushed approach to donor insemination and the vision of preemptive sperm banking centered the male experience and ego. It took some time for established sperm banks to identify and fill what now seems like an obvious role: to provide a menu of options to straight couples in need of donor sperm. It took even longer for physicians to cede control and retire the practice of recruiting their own donors.

Commercial sperm banks adapted to help propagate more traditional families—to replace one man's nonviable semen with another man's viable semen, and in doing so, fulfill the promise of the norm: a husband, a wife, and children—the American nuclear family.

When I was a young adult, it had never once occurred to me that the medical industry could legally withhold services from me or anyone else, that they could say yes to straight couples and no to queers, but in fact they did just that. Most sperm banks and fertility clinics turned away any woman who wasn't conventionally married. Sperm banks weren't made for lesbians.

It turns out lesbians didn't need them. Instead, while sperm banks were growing, lesbians were developing elaborate networks to support each other. The idea that lesbians could become parents on their own terms was, at the time, revolutionary and connected to the larger feminist goal of giving women full control over their reproductive health. Lesbians and allies organized groups for queer women who wanted to become parents, either as partners or single mothers. They passed out instructions on how to perform inseminations with turkey basters, diaphragms, and needleless syringes. They found clever ways to source sperm.

One way completely avoided any doctor's office. Several

mothers of now-grown children have explained to me how it worked in Seattle in the 1980s.

If you were a lesbian who wanted to get pregnant by an anonymous donor, you needed to find yourself a go-between, a friend who would make things happen for you. The go-between would ask around and find a donor—often a gay man in the larger community. The donor could be a close friend, or a friend of a friend, or a colleague from work. The go-between would know him, but he would be anonymous to the recipient.

In these networks, there was paperwork involved: a survey that asked for basic medical and personal history, not unlike the donor files available to sperm bank clients. The go-between collected this and shared it with the recipients. She kept a separate file with personal information—the donor's name, his social security number, the recipients he'd been paired with. In theory, this could be shared with the recipient family when the child turned sixteen, and the family could decide if they wanted to track down the donor and contact him. In practice, this exchange didn't always happen quite like that. Through the course of the interviews I conducted, I heard anecdotes about forms being lost due to illness, death, and human error. However, community and memory are living things, and in some cases, those who wanted to find their donors could do so by simply asking around.

Hopeful recipients charted their cycles with the same tools I used to chart mine: a basal thermometer, a chart, and a pen. When it was time to inseminate, the go-between was the emissary. She picked up the ejaculate (two women mentioned artichoke jars as the container of choice) and kept it warm as she transported it to the home of the woman who was trying to conceive. At that point, the go-between helped, or bore witness, or got out of the way, but her role wasn't just functional—it was spiritual. Her presence conveyed the blessing of the larger community.

Someone who was a go-between once would likely be a go-between multiple times. She would have a list of men who were ready and willing and who already knew the drill.

As I learned about these networks one generation later, I was amazed by their efficiency and how many problems they solved. The network system outsourced the difficult legwork of finding a donor to the go-between, a person who, because she lacked direct personal investment, could more comfortably manage those negotiations. If Kellie and I had employed this approach, and if, say, Dee had been our go-between, then we would never have known the particular torment of waiting weeks for an answer that would never arrive. Jesse could have delivered his no to Dee without feeling the pressure of our hopes. We wouldn't have been hurt by his no, because we wouldn't have even known about it. Instead, we would have simply sent our friend on a mission, and we would have heard back from her once she was successful.

What's more, the network system preserved anonymity

while allowing the would-be parents to rest easy knowing the sperm wasn't coming from an unknown stranger but a community member who had ties to mutual friends. This system was free and spared recipients from having to medicalize the practice of babymaking.

Others have told me stories that capture another mode of conception that was common to lesbians in the '80s: insemination via feminist health centers. These centers—connected to the larger women's health movement—were established and run by women who sought to empower their peers. This was the generation of feminists who got together in groups and learned how to view their cervices using a speculum, a flashlight, and a mirror.

Olympia had one of these centers, founded by a woman whose name is still legendary among locals: Pat Shively. Pat was a lesbian herself and a mother of three children from an early marriage. (It's worth noting that heterosexual sex—often the byproduct of a youth spent in the closet—is the oldest form of conception available to lesbians.) When Pat opened the Women's Health Clinic in 1981, she didn't do so with the vision of helping fellow queers conceive but with the broader mission of serving diverse populations of women. Her clinic offered abortions, and she made herself available at any hour of the day or night to administer rape kits to women who had been sexually assaulted.[8] I imagine that it must have been a small comfort to those women, in a moment where small comforts mattered, to be seen by someone who was capable of hearing and believing them, by someone who knew how to be tender and also how to fight.

Pat's role as the local abortion provider made her vulnerable to death threats, and she took to carrying a Glock and wearing a bulletproof vest.[9] In the photos I've seen of Pat, she has a small frame, short unkempt curls, and she is always actively holding something: a phone, a pen, a small child's hand.

So, while Pat Shively may not have set out to make a clinic for the explicit purpose of helping lesbians conceive—while it may not have even been part of her original vision—it's not hard to see how she wound up filling this niche.

Pat's inseminations were in some ways similar to the informal inseminations that took place in doctors' offices behind closed doors before the era of sperm banks. But Pat Shively didn't have a range of male residents to recruit from. Instead, she looked for college-aged men who didn't smoke pot (studies showed that marijuana use interfered with sperm motility) and paid her donors $30 per specimen. By some accounts, she charged her clients $50 for the inseminations. By other accounts, she did it for free. Either way, it's clear that she wasn't getting rich on the practice.

In this arrangement, Pat acted as both medical professional and community member, a variation on the go-between. She taught her clients how to chart their ovulation and timed the inseminations accordingly. Since hers was a small-scale operation, her donor sperm was fresh, not frozen, and she often performed the insemination on the recipient's sofa.

It is a cruel irony that Pat, who made women's health her life's work, died at fifty-five of ovarian cancer. Her funeral, a friend reports, was packed with dozens of children she had helped conceive. Pat kept records, but they were lost several years after her death when the clinic was firebombed, presumably by antiabortion activists.

In both of these systems—network-facilitated insemination and women's clinic insemination—family-making became a community act not limited to a bedroom or a clinic. Instead, they combined, to varying degrees, personal and clinical elements: the living room couch as the site of insemination, the needleless syringe as the conduit, the friend or partner as the inseminator, the documents that may someday be lost. Both methods centered the humanity of the recipient and allowed her to feel she was the agent rather than the patient.

And, in both of these scenarios, sperm was mainly a means to an end. Between the go-betweens and the recipients, between the clinician and her clients, there was sometimes discussion about what health issues they wanted to avoid or what aspects of someone's ethnic or religious background they might prefer their donor to mirror. Parents-to-be often sought donors who shared their ethnic or religious heritage. But in general, no one had the leeway to insist on blue eyes, or a certain height, or an engineering degree, and it seems that no one obsessed over these details. The attitude that drove these systems was that DNA mattered a little, but not a lot. For the most part, women wanted to make a baby, and they wanted sperm from a donor who was reasonably healthy. That was all.

Contrast this attitude with that of Robert K. Graham, founder of the Repository for Germinal Choice, whose grand plan was to bank the sperm of brilliant men and thus enrich the human gene pool. Graham was a thin man with slicked-back hair and careful posture who was in his midseventies when the bank first opened. He had built a fortune after developing shatterproof eyeglass lenses, but he considered the sperm bank his life's work.[10]

Graham's project might initially sound harmless. After all, if one has to conceive with donor sperm, why not choose a genius donor? Why not offer human evolution whatever boost we can give it? But Graham's vision wasn't based on an innocent appreciation for scientific minds; rather, it was founded on a deeply held ideology traceable to the eugenics movement of the early twentieth century.

In 1970, as sperm-banking technology was advancing, Graham published a treatise, *The Future of Man*, arguing that technological advances had effectively ended the process of natural selection and allowed what he called "retrograde humans" to reproduce at greater rates than their "intelligent" peers. Graham wrote, "As the world becomes crowded with below-average underachievers, we desperately need more achievers," and he offered a set of solutions to that end. Though Graham wrote about human evolution on a global scale, his project was a nationalist one; he was interested in using genetics to give the U.S. an edge toward world domination.

Graham proposed that "intelligent" folks (in the context of Graham's work, "intelligent" is code for white, educated, and wealthy or upwardly mobile) offer society as many children as they could conceive and that society facilitate this by providing youth camps—long-term, publicly funded boarding schools that would spare parents the labor and financial burden of parenting. Graham suggested, "Mothers, liberated from day-and-night childwatching, would then be free to recuperate rapidly from childbearing," and eagerly concluded that this would encourage them to breed more children.[11]

He also proposed that his sperm bank would be one of many, that nearly all urban communities in the U.S. would provide genius sperm to what he called "highly qualified women." Qualified, according to Graham, meant married women of above-average intelligence whose husbands were infertile. In Graham's dream world, heterosexual couples would eventually want to conceive all of their children this way, whether the husbands were infertile or not. Lesbians were, of course, ineligible for these services, and in one instance he told a single white woman that he'd consider allowing her to use the bank if only he could find a way to serve her but legally deny service to single Black women. Nearly all of Graham's donors were white, and Graham was not shy about expressing the reprehensible (and unscientific) view that Black people had lower IQs than white people.[12]

Though Graham's repository may seem like an extreme example, in many ways his practices aren't too different from the system that has traditionally driven commercial sperm banks. Commercial sperm banks, by and large, held on to their policy of serving straight couples until the market—not altruism—demanded they change. Advanced procedures like IVF and ICSI (wherein individual sperm may be retrieved from a low-count specimen), which became more widely available in the late eighties and early nineties, reduced heterosexual couples' demand for donor sperm, and so commercial banks became more welcoming to protect their bottom line. As commercial sperm banks became more inclusive, and as the AIDS crisis introduced new concerns around the safety of semen, the use of networks gradually dissolved.

Today's commercial sperm banks exclude potential donors not just for issues like low sperm count or heritable diseases, but also for height (donors that are five foot eleven and over are strongly preferred, and many banks won't accept donors who are under five-nine) and weight. Gay men, who were so essential to the lesbian insemination networks of the 1980s, are to this day effectively banned from donating at all commercial sperm banks—a policy that is ostensibly to protect recipients from an increased risk of HIV, but makes little sense when one considers that all donors are tested and retested over a six-month period while their sperm is quarantined and that there are no bans on other high-risk sexual behaviors. Straight men can engage in unprotected anal and vaginal sex with multiple female partners and still qualify as donors, while gay men—even those in long-term monogamous relationships—need not even apply.[13]

Most banks actively recruit on college campuses and require their donors to prove that they have earned, or are in the process of earning, a degree from a four-year college, and some banks charge an extra premium for sperm from donors with an advanced or Ivy League degree.

Sociologist Amy Agigian points out that clients are the ones demanding this approach, citing a study where women "placed the highest value on the sperm donor's education, ethnicity, and height."[14] Agigian goes on to point out that any belief that a donor's college education is somehow "transmissible through a man's semen is further evidence of magical thinking about semen that abounds in our culture."

To put it another way, sperm banks aren't simply optimizing their samples for the potential child's future health. They are optimizing to meet demands for children who will conform to societal norms around race and attractiveness. What's more, they are selling a myth that an advanced degree confers heritable traits, that the Ivy League can be encoded into a child's DNA.

Lesbians are now among the consumers driving these demands, and yet I can't help but think back to the early days of lesbian low-tech inseminations and how, for the most part, they were driven not by eugenic ideologies but by personal connections. When it came to alternative insemination, lesbian recipients weren't focused on making genius babies or maximizing genetics. They simply wanted families, reached out for community support, and received it.

I didn't know any of this as I sat on my front porch, holding the Cryobank brochure. I didn't know it, but for the first time, I sensed that Kellie wasn't wrong—that buying sperm was complicated, that it was fraught with ethical dilemmas, and that the story behind the sperm we were getting was actually a story that mattered.

———————————

That night, as Kellie slept, I went online. When I googled "sperm bank," California Cryobank topped the list, and the rest of the first page was filled with companies that looked nearly identical to the brochure I'd already viewed. Their web pages featured chubby, smiling babies, welcomed by straight couples who looked more like J. Crew models than actual families.

I tried variations: "sperm bank small" and "sperm bank gay friendly." I didn't get anywhere. With each search, the same corporations showed up. It was just before midnight when I finally added the word *lesbian* to my search and, bingo, the top result linked to a website that featured a woman, alone, holding a baby. She wore a hooded sweatshirt and a loose ponytail; she looked less like a J. Crew model and more like a person I might actually know in real life. Just above the picture was the tagline: "A trusted resource for women planning alternative families."

Pacific Reproductive Services, it turned out, was a lesbian-centered cryobank founded by Sherron Mills in 1984. Mills, like Pat Shively in Olympia, had been helping lesbians get pregnant out of a community-run clinic. But as demand for inseminations grew, and as the AIDS crisis swelled, Mills wanted an actual donor insemination program that would meet FDA standards—no more fresh ejaculate on demand from a couple of handy donors.

She wasn't the only one. In 1982, the Oakland Feminist Women's Health Center began a sperm donation program that would eventually become the Sperm Bank of California (which, as of this writing, remains the only nonprofit sperm bank in the United States.). And, in an interesting footnote in sperm-banking history, Leland Traiman founded a small operation called the Rainbow Flag Health Services and Sperm Bank, which actively sought to connect lesbian couples with gay male donors. California was a hotbed for alternative sperm sources.

The issue with mainstream sperm banks, as Sherron Mills saw it, wasn't just that they refused to serve lesbians. Mills also believed that lesbians deserved medical care tailored to their specific needs. In a world where the medical model so often assumed heterosexuality, lesbians deserved a place where they could be at the center of the practice, not floating on the periphery.

Over twenty years later, I hadn't known I would need this. I had expected, always, that so long as I lived in a progressive community, I'd be effortlessly folded into the larger system. But here I was, already longing for inclusion, seeking a place that had been designed with me in mind.

As I clicked through the site, I learned that PRS was a comparably small operation and that, besides their alternative demographic, they distinguished themselves from larger commercial sperm banks by offering a catalog of what they called "willing to be known" donors.

"Willing to be known" didn't mean what Kellie would have wanted it to mean. We couldn't take these guys out for coffee and interview them about their life histories and their politics. We couldn't even learn their names. But they did come with a promise—an unenforceable promise—that when our future child turned eighteen, they could access their donor's name and contact information. It struck me as uncomfortable—a little scary, even—that my child upon turning eighteen could make a call and add a stranger to our family. But in other ways it seemed preferable to a closed-door policy, our baby's DNA a mystery that could never be unlocked. My personal stance on secrets was this: I only liked the ones that included me.

I didn't know it at the time, but the "willing to be known" program was a variation on the Identity Release Program, which was developed and trademarked by the Sperm Bank of California in 1983. Today, in the era of DNA testing, all major sperm banks offer a similar open identity option, and many argue that it's unethical to offer donors the anonymous option, since it is likely that any donor can now be tracked down, with or without their consent.

I'm haunted by an anecdote related by Rene Almeling in her book *Sex Cells*, wherein an employee congratulated a sperm donor and informed him that a recipient had recently become pregnant via his sperm. The donor reacted "like somebody hit him with this huge ball in the middle of his head. He just went blank." Later, the donor confessed that he hadn't truly considered the ultimate outcome of his donations.[15] It strikes me that one substantial benefit of an open identity program is that it requires donors to more fully reckon with the end result of their work.

PRS was based in San Francisco where, coincidentally, I would be traveling soon. In just a few weeks, my mother would be attending a work conference there, and I planned to join her to visit a city I'd never seen before and eat good food, walk through neighborhoods, and shop for books.

Oh, and visit a sperm bank. *Is that something people actually do?* I wondered. I recognized the feeling of getting swept up in my own excitement and leaving my level head behind. I tried to talk myself down. There was no reason to make sperm the focus of the trip. Before this moment, I had been looking forward to San Francisco as a distraction from all of this. As I climbed into bed and spooned against Kellie, I could hear my own pulse where my ear pressed against the pillow. People typically ordered sperm online, I told myself, trying to settle my brain towards sleep. There was no real reason for an in-person visit. Certainly I shouldn't let it become the focus of my trip. Maybe I wouldn't even visit it while I was in town.

———————

"I'm thinking of visiting a sperm bank while we're here." I said this within ten minutes of greeting my mother in the hotel lobby. Within an hour, we were searching for the address on a map. She wanted to come too. Her eagerness fed my own.

My mother, when traveling, resembled Big Bird; already tall, she seemed to gain another two inches and hover above any crowd we moved through, taking in the sights with a kind of transparent awe. Like Big Bird, my mother was trusting and curious, and would start conversations with anyone we came into contact with. By this, I don't just mean that she made small talk with the hotel clerk or the cab driver, although she did. I mean that she also sought chances to chat with the family standing outside the native plant exhibit and the couple seated at the neighboring table.

Several years earlier we'd met in San Diego and visited Balboa Park. Outside the pavilion, a large party of bridesmaids gathered and posed around a bride. My mother positioned herself for the best view and watched. I turned and feigned interest in a nearby shrub. When the photo shoot had ended, the bride and her bridesmaids left the pavilion and passed my mother. "Is there a groom somewhere?" my mother called out, the moment the bride came within earshot.

"He's at the chapel," she answered. "You never know these days, right?" They shared a chuckle, while I took another step away from them. I was ambivalent about this trait of my mother's. She made it impossible for me to blend with the scenery.

The sperm bank was less than two miles from the hotel where my mother and I stayed. Together, we walked through a neighborhood of restaurants and bookstores, and then took a left down a hill and descended into a district that was gray and industrial. I kept my eyes fixed on the numbers, and stopped when I spotted the address, 444 De Haro Street, outside a monstrous building built of concrete, glass, and steel. It was a Friday afternoon, and there was no one in sight, though the corridor was vast, with high ceilings and potted palm trees. I felt like an interloper in the corporate world, snooping around with my mother, looking for sperm. I was afraid that a roaming security guard might stop us and ask what we were doing.

But eventually I found it, up one flight of stairs and tucked around the corner. Inside Suite 222, the decor changed dramatically, from bank lobby to massage therapist's office. The hall smelled of essential oils, of lavender and eucalyptus. A long-haired receptionist sat just beyond the entrance and greeted us. In an effort to keep my mom from talking first, I introduced us right away. "I called last week about visiting," I explained. "I've been trying to settle on a sperm bank, and I just figured since I'm in town—"

"Of course," she said, nodding. "You might want to spend some time in there," she suggested, indicating a private room that featured houseplants, a round table, and two wicker chairs with floral-print cushions. "That's where we keep the donor profiles." She explained that there were two special binders that held childhood photographs of every willing-to-be-known donor. Each photograph had a number that corresponded to a profile in a separate binder. "Settle in, take as long as you want, and let me know if you have any questions."

I reached for one of the photo binders first, and my mother took the other. They were wide three-ring binders stuffed with crisp sheets of plastic that shined beneath the light. Each page held two photos, one above the other. On blank sticker labels, someone had handwritten each donor's number. Some of the photos featured newborn babies, red-faced and swaddled in blankets. Those weren't so helpful. Others were school-issued photos from first or second grade. They had big smiles with missing teeth, or corduroy jackets, or Afros.

My mother and I sat side by side, studious. Each time one of us turned a page, there was the soft sound of plastic unsticking. Occasionally my mother would chuckle and tap my arm. I'd crane my neck to view her binder. Her choices were different than mine: boys with tidy hair, bow ties, and sparkling teeth. I liked the boys with the shaggy hair and awkward smiles.

What struck me about the binders was this: throughout my twenties, I'd been paying attention to my feelings about individual children. Though I liked children in general, and though I was sure that I wanted to have my own, there were plenty of kids whom I could take or leave. They were the boys with buzz cuts and truck T-shirts who begged for toy guns at Target or the girls in faux-fur coats belting out pop songs I barely recognized. Certainly these children were adorable to someone, but they sparked nothing for me. There were plenty of adults I had no interest in or didn't connect with. Why should kids be any different?

Then there were the kids I wanted to take home with me, the girl with long brown hair and freckles who leaned off the side of her father's shopping cart. Or the boy with the wide eyes and gap between his teeth who drew pictures while waiting for his food to arrive in the restaurant. As I looked through the binder of photographs, I had an instantaneous reaction to each one. Some of the photos didn't interest me at all, but others tugged at my heart. It may have all been an illusion—a crooked bow tie or a Snoopy shirt may have signaled to me, erroneously, that this child felt like kin. The photographs in all likelihood could not predict how I would have felt about the donor as a grown man. But even if my intuitions were illusions, I appreciated them. The photos gave me a sense of control, a sense that I was choosing a person rather than a number.

My mother lost interest in the photographs eventually and

let herself out of the room. As I pored over donor question-naires that matched some of my favorite photos, I could hear her chatting with the receptionist, explaining that I had a partner, Kellie, who lived with me in Olympia. "You must get quite a few lesbian couples here," she said. When she began offering the details of our lives, I hurried to join my mother at the desk.

As I approached, my mother put her arm around my waist. "I was telling her about your situation," she said. I felt my cheeks grow hot.

The receptionist laid her hands on her desk, as if she had no other tasks to attend to. "Do you have any questions I can answer?" she asked me.

I had just one. I wondered where their donors came from. "Are they all in college?" I asked.

"We get some college students," she said. "But, actually, we advertise on Craigslist. That's how most of our donors come to us."

I let out a laugh. I wasn't quite sure what to do with this information, that the sperm at this clinic came from the place I associated with free couches and unwanted cats. It seemed that I could have chosen to be troubled by this. But, more than anything, I liked it. I liked the idea the donors were invited rather than recruited, that the call for them went out to the community at large.

"We get a better range of donors that way," she explained. She was right—from the profiles I'd looked at, most of them listed actual professions rather than majors; I'd seen a doctor, a fireman, an electrical engineer.

That night, in the hotel room, my mother and I each sat on our own bed, each with a bedside lamp on, reading. As she read the book she brought, I spread open the folder that the receptionist had sent me home with. The files didn't contain much information that was new to me. There was a FAQ page, a handout on how to chart your cycles, and some specifics on shipping and ordering, but I read every word carefully, as if I were studying blueprints for a home I would soon build.

8

DONOR MATCH

When I got home from San Francisco, I printed the catalog of willing-to-be-known donors. As Kellie lay in bed one morning, I delivered it to her along with a pencil and a cup of coffee. My heart raced. "You give it the first look," I instructed. She put on her reading glasses and propped the document against her knees. She looked so studious that I wanted to kiss her, but I held back. If I distracted her from this task, I feared she might never return to it.

The sperm bank offered an intriguing option, a service they referred to as "donor matching." If we submitted our donor short list and a photo of Kellie, an employee would sit down and determine which donor most closely resembled her. Even better, if she found a striking resemblance between Kellie and a donor we hadn't listed, she would redirect our attention to his profile.

There was one woman in charge of the donor matching, and I liked to imagine her in a small, well-lit room with photos of

Kellie and a dozen men spread out across a table. It struck me as a mystical process. I wanted to believe that through her magic she could conjure a stand-in for Kellie: a tall and gentle man with steel-blue eyes.

"Donor Match" became an ongoing game that Kellie and I played anytime we were out in public. It started one day when Kellie came home from work to report that they'd hired a new seasonal worker who looked just like me: dark hair, heavy eyebrows, and hound-dog eyes. If we had needed a donor match for me, he could have been it. From that moment on, I was always scanning my surroundings for donor matches for Kellie. We might be in the grocery store and I'd see a man Kellie's age wearing work boots and polar fleece, reaching for a box of pasta. I'd lean into her ear and whisper, "Donor match."

Occasionally we had interactions that made the near-stranger donor match feel just out of reach. Over the years of working on the cabin, Kellie and I had become regulars at the lumber store on the edge of town, which turned out to be one of the few places in Okanogan County where we felt like we could be ourselves. The owner, Mick, was a tall and handsome man with a neatly trimmed beard whose wife owned the plant nursery next door.

It was Mick who sized Kellie up and sent her down the road to the salvage yard, where an old man named Phil, who was barrel-chested, bearded, and missing two fingers, collected wood that had history. Phil sold us four hundred square feet of fir floorboards that had once been part of an apple storage warehouse and an old wine barrel the size of a roomy garden shed. The floorboards were practical, but the wine barrel was more of an impulse buy. Kellie imagined that she might find a way to convert it into a sauna, and then she quickly fell in love with that dream, and so we returned a few weeks later with two hundred dollars and a flatbed trailer. Phil became our occasional source for special salvaged wood and our regular source for garbage bags of shavings, which we used to keep down the stink in the outhouse.

But sometimes Kellie and I just needed a dozen sheets of plywood or some pressure-treated posts, in which case we dropped by Mick's. Mick had an employee who was shorter than Kellie but could have passed for her younger brother. He had olive skin and sandy hair and wore beat-up work pants with fleece-lined hoodies. He reminded me of a sitcom character; he was goofy and boisterous with an easy, booming laugh. On the afternoon when we bought the wood for the floorboards, the three of us loaded the wood into the trunk together, and when we were done he began fumbling with the pocket of his flannel shirt. "I want to give you something," he said, and he proceeded to pull out a single, perfect marijuana bud. I was embarrassed and flattered. Kellie took the bud and tucked it into her own identical shirt pocket. My cheeks were still hot as we drove away, the air in the cab already thick with bud scent. "Whew!" I said. "Donor match."

The idea of donor matching became a way for us to make peace with the process, a way of making sperm selection seem less arbitrary, less anonymous. We weren't choosing a stranger. We were choosing a match—like a game of memory cards where you turn one card over, and then another, then another, until you find a pair, stack the cards together, and feel satisfied that something is complete.

The process of donor matching was a sign of how far we were from the days of lesbian networks and feminist clinics when the choices were limited, where you more or less took the sperm that you were offered. I didn't think about that much, though. I didn't think about whether or not it mattered if our child looked like Kellie or about what meaning we would make of that resemblance. I simply thought it would be a cool and satisfying trick to bear a child that looked something like my partner. The catalog gave us hundreds of choices, and this was one simple way of narrowing them.

After a few weeks of passing the catalog back and forth, of starring our choices, our top pick was a guy listed as six foot two, athletic, and a Canadian of Ukrainian descent. It was hard to explain why we had chosen him—or anyone on the list, for that matter. We started with medical histories that scared us the least, with features and interests that sounded like Kellie. But once we purchased the long profiles of our top ten choices, we found ourselves scouring pages of handwritten questionnaires. At that point we became less concerned about anything quantifiable. Instead, it seemed that, more than any particular answer to any particular question, the handwriting itself told a story. Overly neat handwriting made me suspicious, like the donor had something to hide. I took comfort in handwriting that was legible but hurried. Also, I noted to the tone with which the answers were delivered. Some of the donors seemed bored or curt. They answered in two words when possible. Some of them seemed overly confident. One of them wrote: I am certain I would be a suitable donor because I have excellent athletic ability and my IQ score is well above average.

And then of course there were the childhood photos. In his photograph, our top pick—the Ukrainian Canadian—had smooth blond hair, combed to one side. He looked about four and was posing for a professional photo with the standard mottled blue background. He was bright-eyed, looking beyond the photographer and grinning. This smile reminded me of a photo I'd seen of Kellie at a similar age. In fact, the major difference between Kellie's photo and the donor's photo was that, instead of a tie, Kellie had been forced into a paisley dress and her hair was unnaturally poufy because her mother had insisted on curling it.

Lisa, the sperm bank employee who took care of the donor matching, agreed that the Ukrainian Canadian was a good fit for us. We talked to her on the phone one afternoon, after she had performed whatever matching magic we had paid her to do.

"Can you tell us anything about him?" Kellie asked Lisa.

"I can't go into specifics," she said, "but I can tell you that these guys come in here week after week and we get a sense of who they are. And we like 396. He's someone we used to look forward to seeing. But I want to make sure you noticed he's no longer an active donor. We've got ten vials left, and when it's gone it's gone."

"Okay," Kellie said. She sounded gloomy. I itched to get off the phone, to place our order before someone else bought all of his samples.

Lisa must have read the hesitation in Kellie's voice. "I know it's a huge decision. But no one has ever met their new baby and then called to complain that their donor was a dud. That's just not how it goes. You're going to love your baby."

After our phone call with Lisa, Kellie stood behind me, one hand on my shoulder, as I placed the order with our credit card. Ten samples. All that was left of our donor. With shipping, the total came to just over three thousand dollars. It hurt me to pay so much when I felt certain that I would be pregnant after one or two tries. Still, I didn't want to tempt fate. I filled my cart. "You okay with this?" I asked Kellie as I entered our credit card number.

"I think so," she answered.

III.

9

A SECRET

The first successful doctor-patient artificial insemination took place in 1884. The procedure was a secret. The recipient, a thirty-one-year-old woman who remains unnamed, was never told what was happening to her—not before, not after. Instead, the doctor in charge of her care, Dr. William Pancoast, laid her on the table for what he called an "examination."

This woman and her husband had sought treatment months before. They had tried and tried but could not conceive a child. Dr. Pancoast had at first presumed the woman's body was at fault. In the exam room, he thoroughly inspected her internally before concluding that all of her organs were functional and clean. She was fertile after all.

Her husband, who was ten years older, reported that he had once suffered from gonorrhea. Presumably, no one asked questions; he was allowed to have a history. His "spermatic fluid," the doctor found, was "absolutely void of spermatozoons." He could not make his wife pregnant.

On the day of the final "examination," with six medical students bearing witness, he laid the woman on the table and gave her chloroform so that she would never know. Together, they discussed who among them would provide the semen for the wife. I imagine them there, six students and a doctor, preparing to take liberties with a woman's body. I imagine them joking, laughing, making little effort to hide their excitement at doing something unprecedented and irreverent. Together, they decided on the student who was most objectively handsome. The reports don't disclose where the student went to produce the sample, but I presume he did so privately, that he returned with a jar or a cup, and that the doctor finished the job with a plastic syringe as the students looked on. I presume that the laughter continued—a giggle here and there, an elbow to a rib, a whisper—up until the moment that the woman was revived and presented to her husband.

Maybe I'm wrong. Maybe they were serious and solemn. But I worry they were giddy, inebriated with their power.

The doctors, in collaboration with an unconscious woman, made a life this way. The student's sperm met the woman's egg. A child was conceived and later born. The woman was allowed to believe that she'd conceived via intercourse—a miracle. Eventually, the doctor told the husband, who chose to be pleased rather than outraged and agreed that he should never tell his wife. One of the witnesses, a medical student named Addison Davis Hard, wrote to a medical journal twenty-five years later, to defend the events of that day as a "race-uplifting procedure," and to argue that assisted reproduction could eventually help replace the world's "half-witted, evil-inclined, disease-exposed offspring" with wanted children of high "mental caliber."[16]

This woman's story, the story of being a body underneath the hands of men, of being used but not informed, is a story many women recognize. It is a story of forefathers, of industry—a story of how women can be pushed to the periphery of their own lives.

10
SHE'S NOT MY MOTHER

"I'm dreading this," Kellie warned me. We were on our way to the reproductive clinic, the only fertility specialists in Olympia. Already they were storing the sperm we'd purchased in their cryogenic freezer. Now, we were driving for an intake appointment so that in a couple of weeks, when the time was right, they could perform an insemination.

"Come on," I said. "This is Olympia." We lived in a town that was rumored to have the highest per capita lesbian population in the world. But I knew no lesbians in town who'd gotten pregnant in a fertility clinic. I had no concrete evidence that this place would know how to handle us.

The waiting room was not what I expected. I had imagined leather couches, warm lighting, and potted plants—the kind of décor that might suggest to a client that the thousands of dollars they were spending was being directed, at least in part, to their own care and comfort.

Instead, I opened the door to find two rows of uncomfortable chairs, outdated wallpaper, and fake plants that frayed at the edges. The reception desk was empty, but Kellie and I weren't alone. A woman in a long dress and bonnet stood watching her two boys play in the corner while her husband, dressed in a collared shirt, pants, and suspenders, sat reading a magazine with one leg crossed over the other. Their sons were dressed the same way. I recognized them as Mennonites; I'd seen other Mennonite families before, not at the downtown library or at the local drug store, but always, remarkably enough, at Costco, walking through the aisles with a passel of children, filling their cart with rotisserie chickens and boxes of cereal. I tried not to stare in Costco just as I tried not to stare now. It was hard for me to understand that someone with two sons already would pursue medical intervention for infertility. Two kids seemed like plenty to me. If you found that a third child didn't come easily, wouldn't you just call your family complete? Or was this longing that followed me now a permanent longing? Would one baby only make me want another?

Neither the husband, nor the wife, nor the sons made eye contact with us, but surely we crossed their periphery and they had questions about us as well.

Kellie sat anxiously, her face hidden behind her long hair. Normally, she moved through the world with ease. Just a week earlier, she'd amazed me when she met me for happy hour at a bar that I normally went to without her. It was the kind of place where the waitresses are notoriously grumpy and you tip them extra to apologize for being a customer. That day the waitress and I had a typical curt exchange, but when Kellie arrived she greeted the waitress by name. "Hey, Annie," she said, sliding into the booth.

"How you doing?" the waitress responded. It was the first time I'd seen her face bear any expression other than a scowl. They bantered for a moment before Kellie ordered a beer.

"You *know* her?" I asked Kellie, awestruck.

"Not really," she said. "We've just both been around for a while."

It would never occur to Kellie to fear a grumpy waitress. It was a rare situation, such as being in a clinic like this one, that made Kellie feel she had to hide.

Eventually, a nurse called my name and led us down a corridor to deposit us in a room with a giant desk. "Dr. Lu will see you in a moment," she explained. "And then you'll consult with Dr. Norman."

We sat in silence for several more minutes. Kellie marked time by tapping her foot.

Dr. Lu entered through a door at the back of the room, and we rose to shake his hand. He was a middle-aged man, broad-shouldered and lean.

"Who's this?" he asked, nodding at Kellie. "Your mother?"

My heart dropped. A bank clerk once, years ago, had made the same assumption. "Is this your daughter?" she asked Kellie as she collected the forms we'd just filled out. We were opening our first joint account together. Kellie shook her head and said, "Nope. Definitely not my daughter." I stood there wide-eyed, waiting for Kellie to finish the correction, but she never did. If she had, we would have had to field the clerk's embarrassed reaction. Instead, the clerk gave a strained laugh and disappeared with our papers. Though it was a fleeting moment, I'd never forgotten it—the shame of being unable say aloud who we were to each other, the icky, sinking feeling of having your lover confused for your parent.

"My partner," I said now. I watched Dr. Lu's face to see if he noticed or cared about his error, but his expression did not change.

"Okay, fine," he said and looked at me. "You carry?"

"Yes."

He took out his clipboard. "How old are you?" he asked.

"Twenty-eight."

"How many times have you been pregnant?"

"Zero."

"You've never been pregnant."

"No."

"Are you sure?" he asked.

Was I sure? I was sitting next to my lesbian partner, the second of only two lovers I'd had in my life. I could not even begin to explain to him how sure I was. Dr. Lu stared at me, waiting for my answer. I looked to Kellie to see if her eyes would mirror my rage. In my mind, the worst-case scenario had never been this dramatic. I'd imagined an office that felt like the real-world incarnation of all of those brochures and websites I'd looked at. I imagined doctors who were welcoming, who smiled at us and treated us like regular patients, but who quietly signaled their disapproval. I imagined they might avoid making eye contact with Kellie or that they'd give us endless forms that asked for the husband's name and information, but I never imagined they'd ask if Kellie was my mother or question my own body's history.

"Yeah, I'm sure," I told Dr. Lu. "I've never been pregnant."

His eyes returned to his clipboard. He kept rattling off questions, and I kept answering them; my entire body was tense as if I were waiting for the right moment to flee. I could feel the same tension in Kellie's body. It was like we were one animal.

The questions ended. Dr. Lu didn't waste any time with small talk. "Dr. Norman will come soon," he informed us while rising with his clipboard. This left Kellie and me alone in the office once again.

"I want to walk out of here," she whispered.

"Do you think we should?" I asked. My heart raced. I knew she was right. We should have flown out of there, hand in hand; we should have torn through the parking lot and driven home. But I felt frozen to my chair.

"I will if you want to," I said, and waited to see if she'd make a move.

This was the one fertility clinic in our town. This place had a file with my name on it. They were already storing our sperm for us—I'd arranged it over the phone. Their rates were surprisingly reasonable. I didn't want to wait another month. And besides that, I couldn't imagine walking out mid-appointment. What would we tell the receptionist? What would the Mennonites think? I straightened my back in the chair and told myself it didn't really matter where or how we conceived our baby. Sure, this clinic sucked. But did this process really have to be magical?

"Maybe this next doctor will be better," I said.

"Maybe," she said.

As we waited, my mind wandered to the cabin. One weekend in June, once the walls had been erected, Kellie and I had arrived with a truck bed filled with rolls of insulation. Halfway through the day, when the sun was bright and hot, Dave-Fred drove straight up our hill in his quad, stirring a cloud of dust behind him. He smoked a cigarette and kept a can of Busch Ice on deck.

"Saw you were here," he said, when we came outside to greet him. He took the last drag off his cigarette and put it out with his boot. "If you don't mind working, I thought I'd finish framing the porch. I could use someone to hold the logs steady."

"Sure!" I said. I was overly chipper, determined to prove that Kellie and I were game, that we weren't like those other city folk, those people who earned six figures and had never lifted a hammer. I wanted Dave-Fred to like us, in part because I sensed that he knew what we were—how could he not?—and that he might have had some views about the gays.

My stance toward Dave-Fred was informed not by anything in particular he'd said or done but by my experience so far in Okanogan County. It was a place where you could count on finding bumper stickers that featured a bald eagle superimposed over a rippling American flag or "Rush Is Right" printed in red, white, and blue. There were few places in the world where Kellie and I felt safe enough to hold hands, and though I often felt our discomfort came from an overdeveloped sense of caution, in downtown Tonasket our restraint felt eminently sound. To imagine holding Kellie's hand at, say, the Junction, Tonasket's main gas station and convenience stop, was to imagine at best a series of dirty looks and muttered insults from the clerks and customers, many of whom had likely lived their lives hundreds of miles from any pride parade or gay bar.

Beyond the probability of judgment, I also sensed a chance of violence. A year or two after we'd bought our property, Kellie and I had once driven down the road to swim at a nearby lake. As we dried off beside the boat launch, Kellie noted a faint stench. It didn't take us long to find the source. There was a log at the edge of the lake where snapping turtles often sat to sunbathe, and on this day there were three of them, shiny, round, and still. Too still, actually. As we approached, none of them jumped off into the water. Instead, we got close enough to see that their shells had been blasted open, and their tender insides were exposed and rotting. Someone had shot them for fun.

Around the same time, we learned from the local paper that

somewhere along the back roads not far from our cabin, a crime had taken place. Three teenage boys, drunk, had driven their car into a ditch and, stranded, hitched a ride with a man who'd been gathering firewood. The man drove them a stretch through the forest roads and then stopped briefly when he noticed that some of the wood had fallen off the bed of his pickup. The woodcutter got out to collect it, and as he bent over, one of the teenagers—apparently driven by nothing but impulse—shot him in the back of the head. The story disturbed me, but it didn't surprise me.

Dave-Fred was of this place. The ranch where he lived with his mother was the place he'd lived for most of his life, and while I believed that his friendliness toward us was genuine, I also sensed that I was on his turf and needed to play by his rules. This meant, I believed, never directly mentioning the fact that I was queer, and it also meant proving I was unafraid of work.

That afternoon, Kellie and I took turns holding log beams upright while Dave-Fred stood on a short ladder and pounded them into place with a sledgehammer. As I held the beam, I watched the concentration on Dave-Fred's face and the force with which the hammer struck the wood. *He could kill me right now*; the thought entered my brain and then played on a loop. He didn't, of course. But I never learned to relax around him.

I felt that same sense of caution now.

Dr. Norman entered the room in his white lab coat and shiny brown loafers. He introduced himself with a soft voice;

his hand, when I shook it, was dry and cold. He resembled Mister Rogers, only taller, stooped, and aloof.

"So," he said, looking over the clipboard that Dr. Lu must have handed to him, "we want to have a baby, and we've agreed that the younger one of you will carry."

Kellie and I nodded. He looked up. "I'm going to write in your chart 'Male Factor Infertility.'" Kellie and I laughed together, assuming he was making a joke. Male Factor Infertility, as in: my partner did not produce adequate sperm. My partner, of course, did not produce any sperm. The male factor was simply missing from our equation. But Dr. Norman didn't laugh with us. He lifted his pen and proceeded to scrawl exactly that. Male Factor Infertility.

There was a long pause that followed, a pause that seemed to hold the distance between us like a puzzle. We were amused; he was serious. Months later, as I lay awake in bed one night, I would finally understand: Dr. Norman had no medical template for us. In order for him to treat us, for him to send us through his system, he had to document us as if we were straight, to offer us a diagnosis. It didn't matter that we were undiagnosable, that, as far as we knew, our bodies functioned exactly as they were designed to. We were coming to him for a service, not a cure. There was no place in his chart for him to simply write "Lesbians."

As it turns out, there's no place on anyone's chart to write "lesbians." There wasn't then and there still isn't. Male factor infertility remains the standard diagnosis for all lesbian couples seeking intrauterine inseminations. It's a term that inserts a man in the equation when there is none. There is no infertile man; there is simply a need for sperm. The distinction may strike some as unimportant, but it reveals the medical industry's insistence on viewing the world through a heterosexual frame. To say that Kellie and I suffered from male factor infertility was to lie a little or to dance around the issue. The refusal of the system to name what is—the refusal to use language that acknowledges queerness—is an action familiar to all kinds of queers who so often hear our partners referred to as "roommates" or "friends," who are regularly misgendered or deadnamed, who move through life with many old friends or family members who know our identities but refuse to ever say them out loud.

Kellie and I left the office that day with instructions to call their office once I approached ovulation. During the car ride home, Kellie and I barely spoke. Instead we looked straight ahead at the road, the crosswalks, the traffic lights; we replayed the uncomfortable moments on a loop in our minds, privately, as if by not speaking them aloud we could erase them.

11

AN EGG IN THE DARK

On a Wednesday morning, as I got ready for work, I untangled a pendant from my basket of necklaces. Kellie had given it to me for my birthday years ago, but I rarely wore it. The pendant was a thick square of plastic inlaid with the silhouette of a swallow swooping down to a nest that held two eggs. This morning, I chose it for luck. I reached my hands behind my neck, unhooked the tiny clasp, and threaded the loop through the ring. Last night, my ovulation predictor had read positive. My body was ready. When I called the receptionist at the clinic, she had told me to be there at three. I pushed Dr. Lu and Dr. Norman to the edges of my mind. I didn't want to think about them. Instead I thought of my eggs inside their dark ovary, the thousands of eggs I'd been born with. I thought about the one egg right now that was preparing to burst. What was coded in that egg? Who might it be? I thought about the sperm that was right now cryogenically frozen, that at three o'clock would be unthawed and spun. The cells would be woken, directed to that single egg.

All day, something in me glowed and burned.

Kellie picked me up from work that afternoon to drive me to the clinic. I held on to my necklace. "What if we had twins?" I asked.

"Huh," she said. I scanned her face for signs of panic but detected none. I kissed her as she entered the turn lane. I remembered the days, years ago, when I used to always clutch her arm as she drove; hers was a body that tethered me.

My excitement dimmed the moment we pulled into the clinic's parking lot. The memory of our prior visit was like a fog—low, thin, and cold. I couldn't help but breathe it. This time, the waiting room was empty, just two rows of chairs. No music played. We waited in silence as the receptionist, her back to us, arranged files.

Minutes later, she rose to usher us into a room, where she pointed me to a blue paper hospital gown that lay on a chair and closed the door behind her. The moment I was naked, I feared Dr. Norman's knock. I feared that he would enter the room before I had a chance to delay him, that he'd bluster in, catch sight of me naked, and that he'd act annoyed with me for being too slow or failing to stop him. Such things had happened to me before. But it didn't happen today. Instead, Kellie folded my clothes as I removed them and laid them on the empty chair beside her. She tucked my underwear between my blouse and my jeans. She rose to tie my gown at the base of my neck. Then I sat on top of the exam table and waited. I marked time by swinging my legs, watching my socked feet move back and forth, listening to the crinkle of the white paper beneath my butt. In my life, I've known no feeling more vulnerable than the feeling of being bare beneath a paper johnny.

Dr. Norman knocked and entered with an assistant I'd never seen. He directed us all as he pulled on a pair of rubber gloves. I was to position my feet in the stirrups and scooch my bottom—farther, still farther—to the very edge of the table, so that I was spread wide and bare. Kellie, he said, could stand at my left side if she wanted, and his assistant took her place by my feet. The assistant was a middle-aged woman with frizzy brown hair and an air of disinterest. There was little for her to do at this point, but I found myself thankful to have an extra female body in the room, as if she were standing guard. It didn't matter that she didn't want to be there; I wanted her there, whoever she was.

"Lots of pressure, lots of pressure," Dr. Norman warned before inserting what felt like an entire gloved hand inside of me. I winced and squeezed Kellie's hand with all my might. I didn't breathe until he was out.

"You have a retroverted uterus," Dr. Norman told me.

"You mean it tilts back?" I asked. I'd heard that one before. I'd heard it for the first time when I was a teenager, the first time I'd ever found myself in this position: legs spread, feet in stirrups, hospital gown. My doctor at the time was gentler than

Dr. Norman. She had kind brown eyes and long, gray dread-locks. She narrated her every move, but still every second of the exam seemed to last minutes. *Your uterus tilts back,* she had told me. *That's true for about ten percent of women.* In that moment I had thought about overlapping statistics. I had just confirmed for myself that I was queer after kissing my first girlfriend while waiting for a bus. One in ten women were gay. One in ten women had a retroverted uterus. That made me one in one hundred. What other unlikely things would I discover about myself?

"Does that matter?" Kellie asked.

"It's not a problem," he replied, "just an item of note." He had already pulled a metal speculum from his drawer. As he inserted it into me, I closed my eyes and tried to think of other things. I thought about being back in the car with Kellie when this was over, driving toward home. I tried to remember what was in the refrigerator so that I might consider what to make for dinner. Nothing good. Maybe we'd get takeout. I thought about my kitchen table, a place where I belonged. I thought about cartons of white rice and salty shrimp and noodles.

Dr. Norman reached for a second metal tool. It looked like a long pair of scissors, only its ends curved into two small hooks. The doctor explained that he'd use it to bind my cervix. If I had not glimpsed the instrument, the tenaculum, beforehand, perhaps its insertion wouldn't have felt so sharp to me. "Lots of pressure, lots of pressure," he whispered, but it didn't feel at all like pressure; it felt like exactly what it was: a sharp metal instrument pinching some part inside of me that was never meant to be pinched. I squeezed Kellie's hand harder, ever harder, and willed myself to breathe. Kellie squeezed back.

Dr. Norman, having finished the insertion, stepped away from me. He peeled the glove off his hand and held it for a moment between two fingers before dropping it in the wastebasket. "I'll be back," he promised. The door swung and closed behind him.

I looked over at Kellie. My eyes were tearing from the pain.

"You okay?" she asked.

I nodded. The assistant looked on in silence.

Dr. Norman returned holding a syringe in his gloved hand. The syringe ended not with a needle, but instead with a slender tube about half a foot long. I knew from my research that he would need to insert this tube inside my os, the tiny hole in the center of my cervix. This was the benefit of intrauterine insemination, the reason we were paying for this procedure rather than simply thawing the semen at home and inserting it ourselves: the sperm would be delivered directly to my uterus. They would not have to navigate the long canal of my vagina; they wouldn't have to find their way to and through the os. Instead, they would be delivered directly to my womb.

Dr. Norman looked intent as he made the insertion and slowly, carefully pushed the plunger, releasing the fluid inside of me. Though my body remained tense, I tried to visualize an opening, a welcoming. Just minutes ago, these sperm had been immobilized, frozen. I imagined that now they were joyous at their reawakening, their freedom, that they swam with determination, seeking my round egg. I pictured my uterus, a home, cushion of tissue, alive with rushing blood, unmarred by metal objects. I imagined one of those swimmers winning the race, penetrating the egg to cause a chemical reaction, a frenzy of cellular division that would someday be my baby.

Though the specimen itself was less than half a tablespoon, it took Dr. Norman a full two minutes to push the plunger into the barrel. As Dr. Norman finally removed the syringe and unclamped me, I felt one last burst of pain as my body began to relax. A feeling of soreness remained.

"I want you to lie on your left side for ten minutes," Dr. Norman instructed before leaving the room, "and then switch to your right. Give the product a chance to wash around your uterus." His assistant followed him out the door.

Alone now in the exam room with Kellie, lying on my side, still in a hospital gown and socks, I laughed and cried at the same time. "That guy's kind of a fuck," I said.

She smoothed my hair away from my forehead. "Are you sure you want to do this?"

"I think we just did."

"I know. But again, next month. We don't have to come back here."

I didn't answer right away. I wasn't counting on another

month. I had already spent years preparing for this moment. We had arrived with all of the ingredients: an egg had been predicted with a chemical test and mobile sperm had been confirmed beneath a microscope. I knew that a typical pregnancy took several tries to achieve. But I knew with a deeper certainty that I was ready, that my body was ready, that my time had arrived.

12

A BODY ALONE

One week later, as I sat in my office grading papers, I felt a sudden and surprisingly specific craving: I wanted a hamburger and a can of grape soda. The thought of what I had actually packed for lunch—brown rice and leftover chicken—made my stomach churn. I warmed it in the microwave and picked at it with a fork. Over the next three days, the nausea grew stronger, more constant and undeniable.

"I think I'm having morning sickness," I told Kellie.

"This early?"

"You think I'm imagining things?"

"I don't want you to be disappointed."

"I know," I said. "But if you were in my body, you'd believe me."

When I drove to work in the mornings, it felt like the sky was opening before me. Stratus clouds lit orange spread low on the horizon. I stopped at red lights, sipped my tea, and felt aware of my skin, newly plump and tender. I imagined a zygote turning, dividing, and growing. When I arrived in class, I stood in front of my students and taught as if all were normal, but I wanted to leap, cry out, or make an announcement. My life, I was so sure, was changing.

And then, two days before my period was due, as I sat in my office eating yogurt, I was seized by a sudden pain. It was sharper than my typical menstrual cramps. As it eased a bit, I pushed my fingers into the painful spot and breathed. I got up to use the bathroom. There was a spot of blood, brown and sticky, in my underwear.

It took two more days of cramping and spotting for my period to arrive in full, and when it finally came, my nausea disappeared. My appetite returned to normal; my period, though, was unusual. I was no stranger to menstrual cramps, but these ones felt not like a dull ache but like a hand reaching inside me and wringing me dry.

I felt foolish for crying, but I did. I curled on the bed in the late afternoon, my head buried in a pillow. Who was I to grieve? I wondered. We'd tried once—once.

Outside the bedroom window, our trees were growing plums. It would be another month before they reached their full size and ripened, but as I looked closely now, I could see on nearly every branch some tiny plums that were shriveling, preparing to drop instead of grow. I took comfort in those plums. I told myself that this was what had happened. My body had made something tiny and inviable, and it had fallen. Perhaps the next one would take shape and grow.

———————————

Failure took on a familiar shape in my house. It began in the bathroom, where, as I approached my period's due date, I pulled down my pants with trepidation, afraid of what evidence I'd find. Sometimes I wore black underwear, half hoping that if I couldn't see the blood, then it didn't exist. But the blood came anyways. It revealed itself at first in streaks of pink on a wad of toilet paper. I tried to convince myself that maybe this wasn't a period. Maybe this was implantation spotting—a sign that an embryo was making a home in my uterine wall. Maybe, I told myself. Maybe this little spot would be the only blood I'd see for months. I willed my brain to imagine this: month after month of clean underwear. It seemed inconceivable, like a feat I'd have to achieve through sheer will. But later, inevitably, my period came in bright red torrents that could not be denied.

Each month, before that blood arrived, I kept an internal list of signs that I might be pregnant: an aversion to the scent of burning charcoal, distaste for broccoli and spinach, suddenly waking at four in the morning. Some of these signs were textbook symptoms of early pregnancy. Others I couldn't find on any list, but to me they signaled a body that was rapidly changing, growing to accommodate a second life.

But my period, always on time, immediately erased these signs and left me to inhabit my body as it was: solitary, lonely.

As I bled, I waited for my next chance.

My hope was tempered by my suspicion that something was wrong. I felt certain that we were successfully conceiving, that every month sperm penetrated egg, creating a zygote whose cells divided and grew. But there was a failure in my body; that zygote couldn't find a place to dwell. It would not implant. My mind carried an image I'd found in my research: that of a blastocyst burrowing into a uterine wall. It looked messy, like it was digging up soft and fertile earth. I wondered what my own terrain looked like: Was it rocky, pocked, and hard? Was there a reason that no embryo could make a home in me?

"I think there's something wrong with me," I told Kellie after every failure.

"These things take time," she answered.

I watched on as Kellie continued with her life. Each morning from our bed, I listened to her making-coffee noises, her lunch-packing noises. I waited for her to return to the bedroom and kiss me goodbye before she left for work and locked the door behind her, just as she'd done every day for years. To Kellie this was life, not limbo. We were a couple who would someday have a baby. She wasn't in a rush. To her there was beauty in not knowing when it would arrive; there was comfort in allowing fate to make the decision.

None of this comforted me. I had trouble concentrating

on anything but our goal. There were some things I could do: I could show up at work and teach my classes. I could grade papers. I could get together with friends and pretend to enjoy myself. I could contribute to casual conversation, though my thoughts were often somewhere else. But there were many things I couldn't do: I couldn't write except to record my spinning thoughts. I couldn't run because I worried I would shake loose an embryo from its tenuous home. I knew this wasn't true, but still I clung to superstition. I couldn't make conversation with Kellie except to rehash the fears I'd been over a thousand times—that something was wrong and we'd never succeed, that I'd live the rest of my life pining for the child I couldn't have.

Our weekend cabin visits—less frequent now that most of the work was done—were the worst for me. Once we completed all the rituals of arrival—making the bed, turning on the propane and the water—Kellie would carry her chainsaw off to the edge of the property and work on clearing fallen wood in a blissful flow state until dusk. I would walk the dogs, tend the fire in the cabin, and then find myself lonely and exhausted with nothing to escape to. Often I lay on the bed in the stuffy loft on top of scratchy wool blankets, falling in and out of sleep, imagining nothing but a blank slate of failure. I'd spend the rest of that weekend trying to pull myself out of that place and into the rhythm of work. I'd make burn piles or stack firewood or walk the dogs to the creek, but I'd only last a little while before the loft bed called to me, and I returned to a hazy half sleep.

On our third insemination visit, I asked Dr. Norman at what point we should worry, as if worrying weren't already at the center of everything I did. His face registered nothing, and at first I thought he hadn't heard me. I prepared myself to ask the question again. Then he put a hand above my hip and pinched at my flesh. I squealed involuntarily—I was ticklish and surprised.

"You may not have enough chub," he told me. "Go to Baskin Robbins."

I said nothing. I was not underweight. I had plenty of chub. But apparently, that advice was all he had for me.

It makes sense to me now. I had made the mistake of assuming that medicine in general, and fertility medicine in particular, would be flexible—that they yielded to the needs of each individual patient, that Dr. Norman—or anyone—would respond to my particular situation. But fertility diagnosis is intractable, and it's based on an assumption of heterosexuality. A couple begins treatment for infertility after a full year of unsuccessful trying. For the average straight couple, this simply means a year of unprotected sex. But a year of heterosexual intercourse—sometimes casual and always free—was different from my situation, my months of charts and ovulation predictor kits, the sperm that had been examined for motility each month under a microscope, the thousands of dollars we had already spent. Every try so far had been expensive and precisely timed. It seemed like a waste to just keep trying for a year, when

I already suspected my body might have a specific and treatable problem.

I would later learn that if I had lived in San Francisco, and if I had gone for inseminations at our sperm bank where the majority of their clients were lesbians, they would have steered me toward fertility testing after four unsuccessful tries. They had developed this protocol because they saw and understood their patients.

But Dr. Norman didn't see or understand me. To him, I was an oddity, a patient who didn't fit in his mold. Instead of adapting his protocols, he more or less ignored me.

To this day, there still aren't any widespread protocols specific to lesbians and other queer folks who are trying to conceive. We show up at sperm banks or fertility clinics and are treated like anomalies in spite of the fact that we are our own demographic with specific needs, needs that might be easily studied, assessed, and responded to. It would be so easy, I believed then and still believe, to simply decide that for people who are tracking their cycles and precisely timing their inseminations, four months can replace the standard one-year guideline.

At the time, I thought that perhaps all I needed was a different doctor, someone who would listen to me explain my experience of my body: every month I had pregnancy symptoms and yet every month I bled on time.

A friend of mine suggested I visit Dr. Xiao, a Chinese acupuncturist-herbalist in Seattle. But acupuncture sounded too subtle to me. I wanted a cure, not a process. Another friend recommended Dr. Robin Tran in Tacoma. She was one of the few doctors in the state who was willing to help women deliver vaginally after having caesarian births with earlier children. If nothing else, Dr. Tran sounded like an advocate, the kind of doctor who might be willing to buck protocol for her patients.

Less than two weeks later, I sat in Dr. Tran's waiting room, filling out my medical history on a stack of pink photocopied pages. Throughout the course of my adult life, I had grown to hate medical forms, with their endless checklists of diseases, hospitalizations, and family histories. Did anyone ever look at these? I spent extra time on the first page of Dr. Tran's form, which asked me for my husband's information. I drew a line through the word *husband* and above it printed, as neatly as I could, the word *partner*. Next to the word, I wrote Kellie's name. I wondered if anyone would see this and take note—the receptionist, maybe, or an assistant. If they noticed, might they gently point to that spot as they handed the paperwork to Dr. Tran? Might they tap her on the shoulder and say, *Just so you know, your next patient is gay?* I wanted to hope that they would. I wanted to hope that the purpose of the paperwork was to save time and spare patients and doctors from awkward exchanges. But experience told me that the form would simply be filed away, and that Dr. Tran and I would be starting from scratch.

In Dr. Tran's office, the window overlooked the parking lot. I could see my own car. It was autumn now, and all was still except for the occasional yellow leaf that floated from a tree. Dr. Tran burst through the door, all energy, and firmly shook my hand. She pulled her rolling chair so that she sat directly across from me, and then she leaned in and looked me in the eye. "It's been a long, hard road, hasn't it?" she asked.

The comment caught me off guard, and for a moment I wondered how she knew me so well. How did she know about the years that Kellie and I had spent in conversation, our months-long quest for our donor, our sense of isolation at the clinic, the last three months of disappointment? How did she know about all it had taken to bring me here? Was it written on my face? Or perhaps, in the minutes I had waited for her arrival, she had studied the paperwork I filled out. Perhaps she had noticed that I crossed out *husband* and immediately understood the world I'd been navigating. "Yes," I said softly, waiting for her to reveal herself.

"So you've tried three intrauterine inseminations," she said, glancing at the paperwork I'd submitted to the front desk minutes earlier. "How long have you been trying to conceive?"

"Just those three times," I said, puzzled by the question.

"Three times?" she asked.

I nodded. "Three IUIs."

A storm crossed her face. She stared at me a moment. "Why on earth would you *begin* with intrauterine insemination?" Dr. Tran's voice was markedly annoyed.

"Because my partner is female?" I said it tentatively, half apologizing. I waited for her manner to shift, for her to realize her assumption and move from annoyance to apology. *Oh, of course*, she could have said. *I should have noticed that on your chart.*

But she didn't say that. She simply continued to assess me through narrowed eyes.

To break the silence, I filled in the details. "I know it's only been three tries," I explained, "but each month I have pregnancy symptoms, and then my periods aren't normal. It just seems like something's wrong."

Dr. Tran let out a great sigh and turned to her computer. I could see only the long, dark ponytail that trailed down her back.

"Have you had a positive pregnancy test?" she asked.

"No," I admitted.

"Most people wait a year," she told me as she typed.

"I understand that," I said. "But I'm paying for every try."

"You'll have to wait like everyone else," she said, and then she reached for her prescription pad. "This is about all that I can do for you right now," she said. "It's a prescription for progesterone." She signed her name with a flourish and then offered me the page. I had to lean in to reach it. She wouldn't look at me.

"What will this do?" I asked her.

"Sometimes it helps prolong the luteal phase," she told me. She offered no further explanation. Instead, she stood up and turned her body toward the door.

"Okay," I said. I paused for a moment to see if she would offer anything else. Was I to come back at some point if nothing worked? I wondered, but I didn't want to ask. She said nothing, and so I left. It was clear she didn't plan to see me again.

I walked to my car with the prescription between my thumb and forefinger. Once I settled into the driver's seat, I examined it, as if I might find an answer there, in the number of milligrams she'd written or in the lines and loops of her signature. Inside the walls of Dr. Tran's office, I'd felt small and embarrassed. Now that I was alone, I felt a tide of rage spread through my body. My breathing went shallow and the edges of my ears burned. My appointment had lasted eight minutes. This was a doctor whom I had been told cared deeply about the women she served. But apparently not me. What I held in my hands now was not so much an answer as it was a token. She might as well have handed me a lotto ticket.

13

STORIES AND MAPS

"Stop taking the progesterone," Dr. Xiao commanded me during our first meeting. I had tried and failed in sets of three—three tries without progesterone, three tries with—and decided that herbs and needles were worth a shot.

Dr. Xiao had a round, freckled face and wore her long black hair in a braid. She had put on a pair of black reading glasses to examine the thick stack of fertility charts I had handed her, all of them crinkled and some of them tea-stained. As she studied each one, I felt a small sense of accomplishment, as if all of the months of logging my temperature finally counted for something. "You worked hard on these," she said.

Dr. Xiao held up my most recent chart and pointed to the line that indicated the second half of my cycle. "You have plenty of days here," she explained. "Progesterone's not helping you." She moved her finger to the midpoint of the chart, the sudden line that signaled ovulation. "We'll work to make this stronger," she said. "I want to see a sharper rise."

I had mentioned from the beginning that my partner and I performed six inseminations using donor sperm, and as I sat there, I wondered if she, like Dr. Tran, would assume that I had a husband, that we'd been trying for a year before moving to a clinic. I braced myself for questions, but either Dr. Xiao understood exactly what was going on, or she didn't care about my partner or backstory. Perhaps the lines on my chart told the only story she needed.

"Wait three months," she instructed. "Don't try. Don't spend your money. Give me time to work."

For Dr. Xiao I kept my clothes on, but rolled my pants up over my knee. It was winter by then, and my legs were unshaven. I lay down on her table, closed my eyes, and pretended to relax. Her office smelled like roots in wet earth—like ginger and turmeric and other medicines I couldn't name. A small fountain trickled in the corner. Dr. Xiao stuck needles in my wrists, my ankles, and my feet. Sometimes she stuck my ears, and sometimes she stuck between my eyes. The points changed from visit to visit, and I wondered how she chose where the needles would go. Did she see different things each time she looked at me? Always, the last thing she did was place a call bell beneath my right hand. "Ring if anything's not right," she instructed.

When she left she closed the door behind her, and I would feel how the needles were shifting things around, opening veins, rerouting blood, stretching my nerves. I knew people who claimed to love acupuncture, who said the needles relaxed them, that they fell asleep on the table and left the office feeling restored. I was not one of those people. Sometimes an ache would move up and down my leg. Sometimes a particular needle felt especially sore, and then the pain would pass. Sometimes my stomach gurgled and turned. Sometimes a great wave of discomfort would travel through my body. The discomfort was never great enough that I considered ringing the call bell. I treated these feelings as the medicine doing its work. But what drove me crazy was the waiting. Sometimes Dr. Xiao returned and removed my needles after only twenty minutes, but more often she left me there for so long that I could no longer track time. I would hear a door open and close, hear her footsteps in the hallway, and think that she was finally coming to release me. Then I would hear her enter another room and talk in muffled tones to a different patient. My stomach growled in hunger. I had to pee. I thought of the piles of student papers waiting in my office sixty miles away. Often I wondered if she might have possibly forgotten about me, if perhaps I should ring the call bell to remind her I was waiting. But I never did. When she finally returned, she set about her work of removing each needle and asking me how I felt. "Good," I always answered.

At the end of the first visit, Dr. Xiao sent me home with a bag of brown powder and instructions for making tea. "Once your temperature rises, you stop," she commanded. "No more tea. When you come back, I'll give you a different tea next time."

I did as I was told. I took comfort in the tinctures, in

drinking each cup until the liquid was cold and there was a sludge made of spent herbs at the bottom. "Are you going to keep that all for yourself?" Kellie teased. I ignored her and closed my eyes. I imagined my ovaries heeding their instruction, my eggs rearranging themselves. They were getting ready in the dark, like bulbs beneath the ground.

I took comfort also in Dr. Xiao's view of things. She seemed to treat conception as an indefinite process, a thing that would take many tries and involve many failures. There would be no instant gratification. So far, she was the only doctor who seemed to honor the complexity of our bodies. Dr. Norman and Dr. Tran had protocols, the same for every patient. Dr. Xiao had herbs, knowledge of meridians, and ideas about my chart. I appreciated that every time I saw her, she sat down next to me and met me at eye level. I appreciated that she asked for my chart every time and traced the lines I'd made. It wasn't just my map anymore; it was hers too.

By the time Kellie and I had inseminated again, our seventh try this time, I had driven alone to Seattle and back seven times. I tried to make luck out of this number—superstition was available to me everywhere—but what I felt more than anything was lonely. After every visit to Dr. Xiao's office, I walked down the street and ate alone at a small Thai restaurant where I was often the only customer. As I pushed brown rice across my plate, I recognized an eerie feeling that had marked my life in different eras, one that I first noticed as a freshman in college. Every weekend, my dorm roommate went home overnight to visit her parents, and I happily claimed our shared space as my own. But though I enjoyed the solitude, I often felt like my own shadow, waking, eating, and dressing with no one to bear witness. Often as I did my own dishes, I sang this line from a Throwing Muses song: "A kitchen is a place where you prepare…and clean up." It seemed like a throwaway line, and yet it haunted me, calling attention to the strangeness of doing something only to undo it, to make a special meal, only to have to do all of the dishes and put them away. Which was, in a way, what my life had now become. All that effort into preparing my body every month, over and over, only to bleed it away.

Try number seven ended in blood.

It was winter by then, and Kellie and I had planned a trip to the cabin with friends. I told myself it was a good thing I wasn't pregnant. Kellie and I rarely made the trip during winter months because snow and ice accumulated on the dirt road. Dave-Fred was under contract to plow all the back roads, but he had warned us that his plow was unreliable, and it seemed that a poorly timed trip to the cabin could result in us being stuck there for days, looking out the window and hoping for the plow.

Even with Dave-Fred's plowing, there were stretches of road so steep that the truck slipped off course. If try number seven had worked, I would have likely canceled the journey. We had heard that there was a foot of fresh snowfall on our hill, and another foot was predicted over the next few days. Being stranded miles from town while pregnant would have struck me as a bad idea.

If there was any benefit to bleeding, it was permission to do things that pregnant women wouldn't. Our friends Laura and Steve followed us in their Civic and put chains on their front tires when we got to our snow-covered dirt road. By the time we arrived, the sky had already darkened to purple, and so we scurried about together, illuminating lanterns, starting a fire in the stove, and piling beds with wool blankets.

Laura and Steve were our neighbors back home. Steve was tall and Laura was short, and they lived with three senior dogs that slept in their bed with them every night. We'd evolved from acquaintances to friends when Steve had set up a propane stove beneath his carport so that he could brew beer, and Kellie dropped by often to smell the hops and watch as Steve stirred the mash. It wasn't so much that Kellie wanted to brew her own beer, but she did want to know how things worked, and so we often found ourselves sitting on Steve and Laura's couch eating pizza and sampling the latest batch of home brew.

For the three days we were at the cabin, we slept and woke to a landscape of snow. Mornings, we bundled up and took the dogs on long, bounding walks, then we came inside to make hot chocolate and devour whatever was handy: tins of tuna and jars of jalapenos on crackers, cans of soup warmed on the stove-top. Every time Kellie and I came to the cabin we left behind whatever dried goods we didn't eat—boxes of mac and cheese, jars of tomato sauce, cans of baked beans. We now had a large enough collection that if we were snowed in, we could comfortably eat for a few days, but not much longer than that.

After snacks Steve and Kellie stayed inside by the fire while Laura and I took turns sliding down the hill on a red plastic sled that we'd bought from the hardware store in town. Though I'd spent my adult life near snow-covered mountains, I had never taken up skiing or snowboarding, and so sledding with Laura was maybe the biggest adrenaline thrill I'd had since childhood. Each trip down the hill brought a real rush—a sense of velocity that was both thrilling and scary. Each time, as Laura whooped at the top of the hill, I tumbled myself off the sled before hitting the ditch, and then I trekked back up the hill with a wide-legged stance, breathless and sweating beneath my gear. It was almost enough to make me forget what I longed for. Almost. And therein lay the problem. Having fun was the best distraction, and yet having fun wasn't a distraction at all. Every fleeting moment of happiness reminded me acutely of what I didn't have. More than I wanted to slide down the hill on a sled, I wanted a child to bundle in winter clothes. More than I wanted to drink hot chocolate on a snowy day, I wanted a child to make hot chocolate for. Everything sweet in life had become bittersweet. Any feeling of joy was tainted by longing.

Try number eight ended in blood. Try number nine ended in blood.

Try number ten was the last try we had, the last of the vials of sperm we had purchased, the last of the samples the Ukrainian Canadian had left at the clinic before moving on to the next phase of his life. My savings account held only five dollars and our credit card balance was climbing. I didn't speak about it to Kellie because I didn't want to face it. I kept my fingers perpetually crossed, kept whispering prayers to myself. Maybe this last try would work.

14

SCREW FATE

All of those stories about infertility, the ones with happy endings, they all seemed to go the same way. The pregnancy didn't happen on the sixth try or the seventh; it happened at some critical juncture, when all hope was on the verge of being lost.

Maybe it happened after three failed rounds of in vitro fertilization, or after a husband learned that his sperm were immotile, or on a mother-to-be's forty-second birthday after half a dozen miscarriages.

A close friend of mine, Victoria, had recently become one of these stories. Victoria was the one who had told me about Dr. Xiao and was also the one that I called each time my period came. She was an easy friend to talk to. Like me, she'd been raised on the East Coast, and so she had a no-nonsense demeanor that was familiar to me. Victoria, with her sensible shoes, tortoise-shell glasses, and head of curls, was not the kind of friend who'd automatically hug you every time you saw her, but she'd listen as long as you felt like talking and crack wry jokes to keep you afloat. Victoria understood like no one else did because she was trying to conceive at the age of forty, and with only one ovary—she'd lost the other to an ectopic pregnancy. She had nearly given up. A couple of months earlier, she'd interviewed with an adoption agency and completed a massive pile of paperwork. She and her husband were preparing to submit a hefty down payment. In fact, I had assumed they had already done this and were preparing for the next step when our phone rang late in the evening. I had settled on the couch with a book and rose to answer the phone before the ringing woke Kellie. I removed it from the cradle and then settled back into my warm spot on the couch.

"I've got news for you," she said. Her voice sounded careful. "It's still early, so no one else should know this."

"Oh my god," I whispered.

Because we were in this together, her good news should have been my good news. "Wow," I said, "this is amazing." I said it from the part of me that meant it. But even before we ended the call, I could feel the weight of my body on the couch. It was the weight of being left behind. Vic and I both knew that this was mixed news for me. I knew that she knew it, and I was grateful she didn't acknowledge it. If she had tried to apologize for her good news, I would have felt even more like an asshole. Instead she said, "You're next."

"Maybe," I said.

I didn't want to be alone, and so I tried to have faith in the happy-ending stories, to believe that my own good news was imminent. I imagined calling all my friends and telling them: *It was meant to be. Our last vial of sperm. Fate was testing us, but in the end it was kind.* My heart lifted as I entertained these fantasies.

But I didn't make those phone calls. My period arrived on time.

There was no special way to mark it, this period that arrived thirteen months after our first attempt at conception. We'd been through summer, then through autumn, winter, spring, and now we were coming to the other side of summer again. I took the dogs on a long walk under a flat, gray sky and thought about what I would have by now if things had gone the way I'd expected: a baby strapped against me, nearly four months old, his warm head nestled against my chest as the dogs pulled me toward home.

I wondered about the eggs that I'd expelled, each one carrying its own unique code of who it might have become if given a chance. They assembled in my brain, a party of babies, all of them wearing onesies, some in bonnets, some in tiny leather shoes, some of them laughing, some of them crying, some of them gazing contentedly at nothing in particular, as newborns often do. These were the kinds of thoughts I entertained every day but never spoke out loud.

My fantasy party of babies connected once more to my hope. It was hope that pulled me through to the other side of each month, and now it was hope that called me toward one more action. When I finished my walk, I would call Dr. Norman and ask him what to do. It was true that so far he hadn't been kind or useful. But now, I realized, we had been trying for so long that we had passed the one-year mark. Maybe he would finally have protocols for us, the same ones they applied to straight couples who'd spent a year having unprotected sex, and maybe those protocols would diagnose my problem. Maybe he could fix me. And so, though it was a Sunday afternoon, I picked up the phone and asked him in a voice mail. We had been trying for a while now, I reminded him. Now we were out of sperm. Should I be taking some tests? Were there treatments I should consider?

His answer was waiting on my answering machine when I returned from work the next day. I could picture Dr. Norman at his desk with his reading glasses on, examining our file with pen in hand. "We normally recommend in vitro after six failed inseminations. As you said, you've had ten of those. So that would be my recommendation. In vitro fertilization."

My stomach dropped. I knew about in vitro fertilization. It was the thing I had told myself I'd never do. For one thing: the money. So far we'd been spending hundreds of dollars each month on our attempts, and those hundreds had added to thousands over time. But in vitro required an investment of thirteen thousand dollars for a single try. It wasn't just that I didn't want to spend that kind of money; I imagined how I would feel that month, in those two weeks leading up to my period's due date. Wouldn't it feel like standing at the black-jack table, having put $13K on an arbitrary number? Wouldn't it feel like watching that wheel turn and turn and turn, not for a minute but for fourteen long days? And another thing: the hormones. It was my understanding that IVF would involve ripening hundreds of eggs at a time, that this ripening would require me to inject hormones every day, and that I would feel chronically tired, weepy, on edge.

Months and months ago, before we'd ever started trying, it had been easy for me to declare that I would never subject myself to this. I believed then that I was fertile. But now here we were. The option was on the table. I was looking at it.

I remembered the time, just after the frame of our cabin was finished, that Kellie decided she wanted a well. She was tired of hauling gallon jugs of water, and tired of accumulating layers of sweat and dust over the course of each stay. I fought her on it, arguing that taking a hot shower at the end of the journey home was one of the joys of our cabin trips. Mostly, though, I didn't want to take the risk. Our cabin sat nearly four thousand feet above sea level, and so it was difficult to predict how deep we'd have to drill. The drilling companies charged by the foot. It was conceivable we could pay thousands of dollars and never hit water.

But Kellie was unswayed by my reluctance, and I eventually agreed but added the caveat that I wanted our property witched. Witching was an age-old practice, more magic than science, where someone carried two metal divining rods over a property and asked them to reveal a water source. When the witcher neared the source, the metal rods, moved by energy, crossed each other. I wasn't sure I believed in witching, but Pat, Dave-Fred's mother, had told us she knew a guy nearby who'd witch our place for thirty bucks. Thirty dollars struck me as a sound investment when it came to choosing a place to drill. If it didn't pan out, at least I could tell myself we tried.

But the man who ran the drilling company talked us out of it. "Nah," he said. "Don't waste your time with that." He had parked his truck twenty feet from the cabin and walked over to an area with a currant bush and some bunch grass. "We drill in this area every day, and we can tell by the terrain where the water is. This right here is your spot." There were plenty of spots on our property with bunch grass and currants, but this one happened to be flat and close to the driveway—easy to access with a drill rig. I understood what motivated him, but I didn't want to make trouble. I agreed to the convenient drilling site.

When the day came for drilling, Kellie made the drive out to the cabin, and I stayed at home in Olympia. I didn't think it would help anything to have me pacing about and worrying while the drillers took care of business. But being three hundred miles away wasn't much better. I waited by the phone for news. Since there was no cell phone reception at our property, I couldn't call Kellie for updates. To reach me, she'd have to drive across the valley to Pat's house or go all the way to town. It was early afternoon when she called. "We're at five hundred feet," she said. "So far, there's only a trickle."

"Shit," I said.

"How far do you want to go?" she asked me.

"I don't know," I said. "What do you want to do?"

It felt like a game of chicken—not between Kellie and me, but between us and the forces of the universe. If we kept drilling, would it all be worth it? Would we hit clear water, or would we wind up spending a small fortune on a thousand-foot hole in the ground?

That's how I felt right now, staring at the possibility of IVF. How much was I willing to throw at this, with no guaranteed result?

Ultimately, Kellie and I agreed to drill to a thousand feet. I held my breath until her next call, which didn't come until evening. She had come to town for a burrito and a beer. There was good news and bad news. The trickle they'd hit at 250 feet was the only water they ever found. But the continued drilling had opened things up a little more, and now we had a thousand feet of storage. Our well yielded an unimpressive quarter gallon a minute, but that turned out to be plenty. Over the years that followed, as we added an indoor sink and an outdoor shower (which was really just an industrial hose with a showerhead hung behind the woodshed), the pressure was fine and we never ran out.

I wondered how we might reach a solution now. In the well

scenario, we actually hadn't needed to drill all the way to one thousand. A little caution and patience would have served us if we hadn't been under pressure to decide on the spot—with a crew of men standing over their equipment and waiting for our answer, there was no time to wait and see. But there were miles between me and Dr. Norman, and I used that space to be skeptical. I had always imagined that there would be a series of steps in between inseminations and in vitro. I had imagined that before they took my thousands of dollars, they'd at least draw my blood and put me underneath an ultrasound. I wondered now if my queerness was once again the issue, if fertility protocols were so rigid, if doctors were so inflexible, that I had no chance of getting the care I needed.

When straight couples entered Dr. Norman's clinic, they paid the same $200 consultation fee that I did. In our case, that fee had paid for a simple "Male Factor Infertility" diagnosis, while for straight couples it launched a series of investigative tests. Men provided samples for semen analysis. Women had blood draws, urine analysis, and ultrasounds.

Dr. Norman had skipped this step for Kellie and me, which was reasonable. We had no semen to analyze, and at the time I had no concerns about my own fertility. But I had trusted Dr. Norman to manage my case accordingly, to decide at some point that it made sense to give me the same workup he gave to any straight, married woman who came into his office after trying for a year.

Instead, it seemed like we had skipped that square in the board game, and going back was inconceivable to him. He'd given us our diagnosis. Male Factor Infertility. We'd already exhausted the limits of his curiosity.

"What's in vitro?" Kellie asked me later in the evening when I relayed the message to her.

"That's the thing where we pay them a million dollars, and you help me inject hormones into my thigh every day. Then they harvest a bunch of my eggs and make embryos in a petri dish."

"Oh," Kellie said, unfazed. "We're not there yet."

"But what then?" I asked her. "What are we doing?" Kellie already knew how I felt about our sperm situation. Even if I could remember our other top candidates from last year's catalog, it seemed unlikely that they'd still be available. And nothing in me felt excited the way I once had about printing out the dozens of pages of donor IDs and basic information. The thought now of combing through each entry with a pencil in hand just made me tired.

"Look," she said. "We'll take another break. We'll figure it out." I didn't believe her, but I was grateful for her confidence. "We'll figure something out," Kellie told me. "It will happen when it's meant to happen."

"You don't know that," I said. I no longer believed in the inevitability of happy endings.

"Yeah," she insisted, "I do. We're just going to take a month or two off. We're going to hike in the desert, come home, and figure this out."

Some weeks earlier, on one of winter's dreariest days, Kellie had convinced me to buy tickets to New Mexico so we could walk under a different sky for a while. We charged it to the credit card. It wasn't much compared to what we'd been paying for sperm. I knew it was a good idea, and I couldn't say out loud the reason I was hesitant: What if I was pregnant by then? I wondered this as I stared at ticket fares. Would I enjoy the vacation? Would I want to leave home? I imagined that any pregnancy once achieved would feel tenuous and that airplane travel, hiking, and sleeping in an unfamiliar bed might feed my anxiety. Instead of looking out to the sky, I'd be checking my underwear for traces of blood. But now, it turned out, the trip was well-timed. We would leave in a week. My period would be over by then. Because we'd be skipping the next cycle, my longing would carry less urgency. In New Mexico, I would simply pretend that I lacked nothing. I would be a woman in the world, whole in my body.

"Okay," I told Kellie, and I filled my mind with landscape, with red dirt and sage brush instead of eggs and tubes and motile sperm.

A few days later, as I looked for shampoo in the grocery store aisle, I ran into an acquaintance. I knew Sarah from the two years she'd spent dating a friend. She had short spiky hair, wore silver jewelry, and when she spoke she often sounded like she was addressing a child. Though we'd spent some time together at dinners and on camping trips, I'd never dropped my guard with her. Her cheerfulness made me suspicious. She and the friend had broken up just as Kellie and I had started trying, so she knew about our plans. "What's happening with the baby thing?" She stage-whispered it with one hand cupped around her mouth.

I answered her honestly. "We're taking a break," I said. "We've been trying for a year."

The moment I stopped talking, Sarah jumped in. "Well, maybe you just weren't meant to be a parent, did you ever think about that?" Her tone was every bit as enthusiastic—chirpy—as it always was.

"Yeah," I answered, nodding, as if she'd said something entirely normal and appropriate. "I've thought about that."

It wasn't until I walked away that I started to hate her a little bit, the way that I hated everyone who acted as if my body's failures were just some feat of cosmic wisdom. For the rest of my time at the grocery store, I replayed her comment in my mind. I wasn't meant to be a parent—because of course, as everybody knows, pregnancy only happens to those who are ready. It happens to those who pass fate's strict test, those who prove themselves emotionally capable, financially solvent, to those who are generally perfect. According to Sarah, fate had deemed me wrong.

I would continue to stew over this comment long after the exchange. Part of me wished I had told her to fuck off, but the other part of me was glad that I had spared her the full spectrum of my anger. Because in the end, all of those voices—the friends who told me to relax, the ones who told me it would happen when I was truly ready—they were just trying to offer anything they could. They were trying to help, and in their trying, they couldn't see that it was senseless—it followed no logic, no order—and that senselessness is the very thing I needed recognized. I needed my friends to say: *There is no reason this is happening to you.* I needed them to say, *Look at you. You're doing everything right, and still it isn't working.*

———————

I thought about adopting. It was an option that I had long wanted to believe was straightforward, convenient, and available to anyone who wanted a child.

Why don't they just adopt? This was a sentence I'd heard tossed about any time a couple had trouble conceiving.

Throughout my lifetime, when I'd thought about my future as a parent, I'd had a similar thought. *If I can't get pregnant easily, I'll just adopt.*

Just adopt, as if it were the equivalent to walking into your local animal shelter, filling out a form, and writing a check for forty dollars. All those unwanted babies. Just open your heart and they're yours.

Part of me still wanted to believe it was simple like that. If Kellie was willing to make the leap and love a child who didn't share her DNA, then surely I could do that too. I didn't need to be pregnant—I was curious about the physical experience of pregnancy, but I didn't long for it. What I longed for was a child. When I imagined skipping the morning sickness, the stretching, the waddling, the water retention, I felt more relief than loss.

I worried a little about the price. I understood that adoption cost far more than what we'd been spending on sperm and inseminations, more than what it would cost to try in vitro fertilization. Still, thirty-five thousand dollars for a baby seemed like a reasonable investment—more than a used car but less than a house.

But then there were issues that I'd only recently started to consider. Adoption had always been framed for me as an act of selflessness and generosity, but what if it was far more complicated than that?

International adoption as we know it began in 1954 with an evangelical Christian couple named Harry and Bertha Holt. The Holts, the story goes, viewed a documentary film on children who'd been conceived during wartime unions between American soldiers and Korean women during the Korean War. Many of these children, who were biracial and born out of wedlock, were scorned and abandoned to orphanages. Moved, the Holts sent aid but then decided they were called to go even further.

At the time there was no legal structure in place to facilitate international adoption, and so, as Harry Holt traveled to Korea, Bertha Holt lobbied Congress, who would go on to pass the Holt Bill, thus enabling Harry Holt to work with the Korean government and bring eight children home. The Holts already had six biological children, so they became a family of sixteen.

Photographs and news reels of Harry Holt surrounded by babies made for good human interest reporting, and soon the Holts were receiving thousands of letters and fielding requests from other Americans wanting to adopt. Harry Holt began traveling back and forth to Korea to facilitate adoptions by proxy, meaning he would obtain children from Korea and accompany them to the United States, where they would be placed with a married Christian couple.[17]

The requests were so numerous that the Holts began "having trouble finding the little ones" in need of adoption, and so their effort expanded beyond placing biracial wartime babies and included full Korean children as well.[18]

The work of the Holts can be assessed through multiple lenses. According to one view, they were heroes, two people moved by faith to offer care and love where it was needed. Before the Holts began their movement, transracial adoption was largely unthinkable. Domestic adoptions were carefully curated so that children appeared to match their families racially and pass as biological kin. The Holts, some have argued, embraced the idea that love transcends racial boundaries.

But if one digs a little deeper, one may take a darker view. Though the Holts referred to the children they placed as "orphans," most of them had a living mother and an estranged father. According to one source, as demand for adoptees exceeded supply, Harry Holt began to coerce mothers into giving up their babies.[19] The Holts were operating with a set of Christian values that one might connect ideologically to the concept of the "white man's burden," the idea that members of the white race were bound to lift up those of other races.[20]

In other words, the Holts were likely not too concerned about how they acquired their children because they assumed that removing a child from a life of poverty and stigma was both God's will and a blessing for the child. In a recruitment letter, Harry Holt wrote, "We would ask all of you who are Christians to pray to God that He will give us the wisdom and the strength and the power to deliver his little children from the cold and misery and darkness of Korea into the warmth and love of your homes"—a statement that suggests that the Holts might have, if they could have, placed *all* Korean children with Christian families in the United States.[21]

The concerns I raise here regarding the Holt legacy remain relevant to international adoptions today. Since 2004, rates of international adoptions in the United States have steadily declined, in part because of widespread corruption. In 2000, the UN published a report on child trafficking in Guatemala that asserted, "It would seem that in the majority of cases, international adoption [in Guatemala] involves a variety of criminal offenses including the buying and selling of children, the falsifying of documents, the kidnapping of children, and the housing of babies awaiting private adoption in homes and nurseries set up for that purpose."[22] Eight years after this report was released, Guatemala closed its program. In 2011, Chinese parents accused government officials of stealing babies and selling them to traffickers.[23] Estimates on how many children were trafficked each year range from tens to thousands. China has since greatly restricted their adoption program, in part because of this bad press, but also because demand for domestic adoptions within China has increased.

Some assert that the number of children worldwide who are obtained illegally is very small and that the decline in international adoptions has dire consequences for the world's orphans. But it's worth noting that people in the adoption industry use the word "orphans" as loosely as Bertha and Harry Holt did. Many children are placed in orphanages as a stopgap measure when a family finds itself in a desperate situation, and many do so expecting to be able to retrieve the child once their circumstances improve. David Smolin, a leading expert on adoption policy, writes, "It is ethically questionable to spend thousands of dollars (or tens of thousands of dollars) to arrange an inter-country adoption, when aid of less than a thousand dollars would have kept the child with their birth family."[24]

And yet, Jane Aronson, founder of the Worldwide Orphans

Foundation, warns that curtailing international adoption does nothing to protect the children who have been genuinely abandoned. Aronson proposes that "if we educated women abroad and showed some respect for their process, we might find that some women would still opt for their children to be adopted."[25]

If one accepts that on one hand there are children who legitimately need care and, on the other hand, the adoption industry often favors the needs of adoptive families at the expense of birth parents, how does one proceed?

And this question became yet more complicated once I factored in my queer identity, because international adoption was and remains largely inaccessible to gay couples. Sending countries set the regulations for who can and can't adopt, and most countries insist on married couples. At the time, the word "married" automatically excluded me because my marriage wasn't federally recognized. Today, though I'm legally married, the word is still code for "straight," since most sending countries don't recognize my marriage as legitimate. Colombia and Brazil are currently the only two countries who officially adopt to same-sex couples. Historically, prospective queer parents have sometimes worked around the system by applying to adopt as individuals from countries that permit single-parent adoptions, but doing so requires an upfront investment of time and money in a process that might end badly if the applicant's identity is discovered, and actively hiding in the closet comes with significant emotional cost.

An open domestic adoption would be, at first glance, more straightforward. Kellie and I would need to attend a day-long orientation, and we'd arrive sweaty and nervous about how the facilitator and the other couples would respond to us. If we were lucky, maybe we wouldn't be the only queer couple. What I worried about more, though, was what would come after. We'd have to create a detailed profile of ourselves and wait for someone to choose us. Us: two lesbians of moderate means. I imagined our profile nestled in a binder dominated by straight couples with six-figure incomes, who could offer their future child riding lessons, private schools, vacations in Europe. I imagined waiting, and waiting, and waiting.

Finally, there was the option of adopting through foster care. Many adoption and foster care agencies are run by faith-based organizations, some of whom have traditionally refused to work with same-sex couples and transgender people. This changed in 2016 when the Obama Administration implemented a policy that withheld federal funding from agencies that discriminated on the basis of gender identity and sexual orientation. This, it appears, was a temporary fix, as the Trump Administration is currently preparing to revoke this policy.

Washington State, however, according to the Movement Advancement Project, was "silent" on the issue of LGBTQ foster parents, meaning that there was neither an official policy to deny my rights, nor one to protect them.[26] We could, if we chose to, begin the process of training to become foster parents.

We could enter the system, report to various caseworkers, and hope for a match that might ultimately lead to adoption.

There was nothing simple or straightforward about any of the above scenarios. To give up on the project of trying to conceive a child biologically and "just adopt" would not simplify my life or guarantee that I'd soon become a parent. And every adoption scenario would require us to subject ourselves to bureaucratic scrutiny. After months of having Dr. Norman reach inside of me and poke at me with metal instruments, nothing in me wanted my entire life examined by outsiders.

———————

The Sunday before our departure, my bed was covered with piles of clothes, my suitcase on the floor as I tried to decide what I would pack. So far, I'd packed two pairs of jeans, one pair of shorts, and five T-shirts. I was happy to leave behind the paraphernalia that had been ruling my life for the past months: the basal thermometer and the ovulation predictor kits, the sanitary pads and the tampons. But just as I was stuffing a rolled-up pair of socks into my hiking shoes, I felt an inexplicable drip between my legs—inexplicable because my period had ended days ago and I was still a week away from ovulating.

In the bathroom I discovered a small spot of blood, the kind of spot that would have been normal if my period had just arrived. To bleed twice in a month was unprecedented, and so I did something equally absurd: I took a pregnancy test. I had a stockpile of them in the bathroom cupboard because they helped me spread out the disappointment of my period. Some months, when the anticipation of my due date was unbearable, I would take a test. When the result came back negative, I knew to expect blood. But this time, for the first time, I could make out a clear double line that indicated a pregnancy.

I wondered if there was any way that I might actually be pregnant. I wondered if some people had periods during the first months of pregnancy or if some stray ball of living cells might have survived the flush of menstruation and had just now decided to make a home in me. Google confirmed that vaginal bleeding during pregnancy was not unheard-of.

I tried to believe that I might be hosting some kind of miracle, while another part of me hovered in judgment. *That's pathetic*, I told myself. *You are having a miscarriage. Not even a real one.*

I added a package of sanitary pads to my travel bag and decided that the next two days would reveal the truth. If I continued to spot and not bleed, then maybe I was growing a baby. But if I began to bleed in full, there would be no reason to hope. I did not disclose my crazy hope to Kellie. I simply complained that our vacation would include the inconvenience of my blood.

Madrid, New Mexico, was a kind of alternate universe, a small town with red hills and a wide blue sky. A two-lane highway ran through the town's center, which included a collection of coffee shops, a pizza place, art galleries, and a tavern called the Mineshaft. Madrid was originally a mining town, and in the hundred or so years since the mines had closed, both everything and nothing had changed. Everything had changed in that the miners had left forever. Nothing had changed in that, when the hippies and artists moved in, they didn't tear anything down or build anything up. Instead, they reshingled the mining cabins, installed indoor plumbing, and hung Tibetan prayer flags on the porches. There were no billboards anywhere, no buildings higher than an average house, and if you wanted to make a phone call, you either had to use the pay phone outside of the pizza place or tilt your cell phone toward the sky and hope for reception.

Kellie and I rented a small casita on the edge of town, owned by a sculptor and a painter who lived on-site with their child. On our first morning there, Kellie wandered down the hill to snoop around the sculptures and piles of scrap metal that lay just outside what appeared to be the couple's art studio. I drank my coffee in the sun, happy for the quiet, happy to be together but separate. The casita sat on one side of Highway 14. On the other side was a hillside scarred from mining: all gob piles and cables and abandoned machinery.

I had finished the last sip of my coffee when Kellie hollered for me. She'd already made friends with the sculptor, and now we were invited inside their home for a tour.

Blinding sunlight streamed into the sculptor's living room, where his four-year-old daughter sat on the floor assembling a puzzle. She had blond hair that was still matted from where she'd slept on it, and the tangles caught the sun. I could see into the kitchen, where the painter, who was married to the sculptor, stood barefoot on the wide-planked floor. She seemed to be concentrating on a recipe, or the newspaper, or whatever it was she had spread across the counter. It wasn't until my eyes wandered to the dark corner of the front room that I saw it: a giant metal crank, attached to a drum—an old industrial winch.

"This used to be the winch house," the sculptor explained. "This place was a disaster when we bought it. This winch was the only thing left standing." He turned the crank then, and the drum rolled smoothly. The giant cable loosened a bit, until the sculptor turned it in the opposite direction. I stepped closer, wondering if I would see daylight in the half-inch crack beneath the winch and the floor. But I only saw space, dark and empty. I was too shy to ask, but I wondered what used to happen here. I pictured coal moving underground in carts, through tunnels, then finally being pulled up here to daylight. And now that the earth had been exhausted, the tunnels were abandoned. The winch was a relic, functional but obsolete. And also loved. That a couple had built their family here, their home, on top of a scar in the earth—that they had turned it into something so bright and beautiful made me ache.

I bled in Madrid, bright red blood that came steadily. I waited for the flow to taper as it would have with a normal period, but instead it persisted. On the fourth evening of our trip, Kellie and I walked along a trail that cut into the desert hillside. The trail had once been a railway, but the coal cars had long ago stopped running along the tracks, and now it allowed us to walk the length of the town at dusk, to look out over the cluster of roofs as the sky changed and the air cooled. These were the moments when my body let go of expectation. It was enough to feel the air against my bare arms.

But as we neared the end of the trail and descended into town, I felt a new gush of blood. By the time we hit Main Street, that blood had spread well beyond my underwear. I could feel it against my thighs and in the fabric of my shorts. Town was quiet except for a few couples sitting outside at café tables.

"I can't believe how much I'm bleeding," I whispered to Kellie. All afternoon as we'd hiked in the Cerrillos Hills State Park, I'd ducked behind shrubs or abandoned mines to change my pad and stash the rolled-up wad of trash in my front pocket. I had packed four pads in my purse and assumed that two of these were overkill, but now I was completely out.

"Are you worried?" Kellie asked. A flash of concern crossed her face.

"A little," I admitted. I imagined myself waking in the middle of the night to a literal puddle of blood spreading far beyond the width of my body. We were far from home, and I had no idea where a hospital was. Also, I thought of the owners in the winch house. I didn't want to leave them with an extraordinary and intimate mess.

"Maybe you should call the clinic," Kellie suggested.

"Dr. Norman won't care."

"We pay him to care," Kellie pointed out. She shook her head. Her worry for me quickly metastasized into disdain for Dr. Norman.

I didn't want to call from the town center, so Kellie and I walked the half mile to the casita and I scrambled up the desert hill, tracking the bars on my phone. The sun had gone down, and the sky was now a dimming purple-gray. I found a reliable spot next to a large prickly pear cluster, and I crouched beside it to dial. The recorded voice instructed me that in case of an urgent concern, I should leave a message and wait for Dr. Norman to return my call. I described my bleeding into the receiver, hung up, and waited. The flow of blood had paused, but I still hadn't dealt with the spill now settling into the fabric of my shorts. Sweat from earlier in the day had dried on me, and I was beginning to feel cold. I wanted a shower. I wanted to wash it all away.

I wondered how long I would wait here. In the casita below me, Kellie had turned on the light and was likely opening a bottle of wine and starting a pot of water as I'd asked her to do. Farther down the hill, the lights were on in the main house as well. I imagined the sculptor and the painter and their four-year-old daughter sitting at the table to eat, passing striped bowls with wooden serving spoons. On the morning of our arrival, the daughter had barely looked at us; she had been content in her play and uncurious about the new adults passing through her home. I hadn't seen her since, but I imagined now the sculptor reaching with his long arms to serve his daughter, to feed her. I imagined the painter, his wife, rising to clear the table, and I imagined this family beginning their ritual for bedtime, a ritual centered on caring for its youngest member. I craved that kind of focus. My days, especially the recent ones, had felt so achingly aimless.

My phone rang, and I answered it. Dr. Norman announced himself. "You're having a miscarriage," he told me. I'd known this for days, and yet I felt relief in hearing it spoken by a doctor. But Dr. Norman didn't pause for my reaction. Instead, he instructed me to seek medical care if I bled through a pad or tampon every half hour. Pad or tampon. Though he'd assessed the tilt of my uterus with his gloved hand, and though he'd prodded at my cervix with the tip of a syringe, it surprised me to hear him mention these intimate objects.

"I'm in New Mexico," I said. In my message, I had explained I was on vacation, but I wanted to make sure he understood. "So I should find an ER if I start bleeding that much?"

"Every half hour is the guideline," he repeated. "Otherwise you're fine."

I hesitated before hanging up, as if he might offer something more. Instead I heard a click.

I hated him. Or maybe I just hated that I was dependent on him—an uncaring stranger—to help me realize my dream of a future family.

I tucked my phone in my pocket and looked out at the sky. The first stars had appeared. Dr. Norman had said I was "fine" and though I resented his indifference, his assessment—from what I could tell now—seemed accurate enough. My bleeding had peaked with the heat of the day and with the motion of hiking. But the gushing had ended. It wouldn't return.

———————

On our last morning in New Mexico, I sat outside again with my coffee. The morning air was cool, but the sunlight warmed me. The wasted hills were familiar to me by now. As I looked out at them, my future spread before me: blank. In that blankness, for the first time in a long time, I found comfort rather than despair. The feeling surprised me.

I assessed the things I knew for sure: I knew I didn't want to see Dr. Norman anymore. I knew that I didn't want to pay money for sperm from men I'd never met. I knew that I still wanted to have a baby.

I assessed the things I didn't know: I didn't know what was wrong with my body, why it rejected, month after month, the cluster of cells that might have grown into a child. I didn't know where our sperm would come from if not from a catalog. I didn't know for sure that I would get the thing I wanted.

For once in my life, for that morning at least, I was okay with not knowing. Maybe I didn't believe in fate anymore, but I found myself nurturing an impulse to move forward, to let go of the things that didn't serve me, to create room for the things that would.

IV.

15
THE MEANING OF SOON

When I told Dr. Xiao about my miscarriage in New Mexico, she thought it was happy news. She laid my most recent chart on the table between us and traced the line that indicated ovulation with her finger. "You're getting close," she said.

I wanted to believe her, but having a miscarriage so early that I mistook it for a period didn't seem like much of an achievement. If anything, it was a more alarming failure. "You'll be pregnant soon," she assured me.

I understood that "soon" was a relative term to a doctor who, all day long, pressed needles into women who were desperate for a child and getting older by the minute. From her vantage, *soon* didn't mean this coming month or the next one. *Soon* simply meant that she didn't expect to see me forever. I wondered if there were things she knew from her years of observations. I wondered if, just based on her initial consultation, she could predict who would eventually conceive and who would give up after years of trying. Maybe it was the women who had already hit forty whom she worried about, or the women whose charts revealed no clear sign of ovulation. Were there women for whom, perhaps, she simply hoped to aid a miracle? And were there women like me for whom the road was mysterious, but it was clear that eventually we'd arrive?

That afternoon, as I stood at the reception desk and wrote a check, a woman my age appeared at the door and struggled to enter while managing the heft of an infant car seat. Dr. Xiao brightened and left her desk to help her. Once inside, the woman placed the seat on the floor and unbuckled her infant. She lifted her baby, who was awake and bright-eyed, and arranged him so that his head nestled in the crook of her arm and Dr. Xiao could peek at him. "I just wanted to thank you," she said.

Dr. Xiao played with the baby's feet. "You made a beautiful boy."

The woman was suddenly unable to contain herself. She sniffled and cried and then laughed. My own eyes teared too. All at once I felt joy and deep jealousy.

I tore the check out of my checkbook and left it face down on the counter. To leave Dr. Xiao's office, I would have had to walk between the two of them or ask them to move, and so I backtracked to the bathroom where I peed and washed my hands and splashed cold water on my face.

I looked in the mirror. I'd been twenty-seven when I decided I was ready for a child. Now I was thirty. I didn't feel old, but

I was disappointed. All my life I had assumed I would get to choose exactly when and how I would become a parent. I had assumed about this, and perhaps in general, that I had more control over my life than I actually did, and I was starting to suspect that there was comfort to be had in letting go.

At home, two uneventful months passed. I was surprised by how it quieted me this time, this measured distance between me and my dreams. It seemed that I could chew my food and taste again; I could breathe in and out again; I could read a book without my mind wandering. When we went to the cabin, I could sit among the aspens and wait for the woodpeckers to reveal themselves, and for the moment, life felt rich enough. We whispered to our closest friends that we were looking for a community donor. We were relaxed about it this time; we didn't make lists or exhaust ourselves trying to come up with new options. We simply hoped that someone might appear.

Victoria, who had entered her second trimester, was one of the friends I confided in. At the end of one of our weekly walks, as our dogs led us off the park trail and onto the main road, she made an offer. "You know, you might consider Dave as your donor." Dave was Victoria's husband. Though I'd never talked to him directly about our situation, I assumed that Vic had kept him in the loop. "I can't speak for him," Victoria said, "but I think he'd be willing. And I would be willing."

I thought about Dave and the first child that he and Victoria had conceived, who was now four years old. Ruby was the first baby to arrive in my circle of friends. Watching Ruby grow from a baby to a toddler to a child had shaped my adult understanding of what it meant to be a parent. We still kept a Christmas card on our refrigerator that featured Ruby at seven months with wispy dark hair and a bright smile. I tried to imagine having a child that would be Ruby's biological half sibling.

"But you know you'd be stuck with us forever," Vic told me.

"That doesn't worry me," I said. I already saw Vic as a permanent friend. But, then again, I wasn't sure I wanted to subject our friendship to whatever surprising feelings sharing her husband's sperm might bring up. When I reported the possibility to Kellie, she said, "Huh," and that was all. We neither dismissed nor pursued the offer. Instead, I slipped it into my back pocket, a kind of talisman to ward off my anxiety.

And then one day, our friend JoAnn came to our house for dinner. JoAnn had known Kellie for about twenty years, ever since they had fought forest fires together on a summer crew. Jo was regular fixture at our house. She watched our dogs when we left town, knew where we hid the spare key, and often let herself in to use the bathroom or get a drink of water if she was riding her bike across town. Jo was short and blond and rode her bike everywhere. She worked as a nanny, and so once in a while she'd drop by with a kid and let him run around in our backyard. On this night, we hadn't eaten yet, but the salad had been made, and we were sitting around drinking wine while a chicken baked in the oven.

JoAnn broached the subject of our babymaking efforts cautiously. This was something I had appreciated about her company. I had one friend who asked eagerly if I had news for her every month. Other friends avoided the topic altogether. But Jo had lost her own tiny son several weeks after he was born prematurely. This was long before I ever met her, but the story followed her. Jo had never told me her story directly, but she alluded to it occasionally, assuming that our mutual friends had filled me in. I believe this is why Jo knew to be delicate. She lowered her voice when she asked, "How's it going?"

I glanced at Kellie. "We're on a break. And we're out of sperm."

"Know anyone?" Kellie asked, half joking.

Jo paused and reflected for only a moment. "Why don't you ask Daniel?" she offered, simply, clearly, as if the solution had been right there all along.

Kellie and I swiveled our heads in unison and looked at each other. Kellie said what I was already thinking: "That would be perfect."

Daniel was Jo's close friend, not ours, and because he didn't appear in our world very often, we had never thought to include him on our list of possibilities. But we had met him twice. We knew that we liked him. We liked him a lot.

The summer before, I had come home from work one day to find a tall man in my backyard, sitting in a lawn chair, deep in conversation with Kellie. His face was shaded by a baseball cap. *Random dude in my yard*, I said to myself.

I continued on toward the back door, where I found JoAnn sitting on our back porch. She was with someone: a tall blond woman who wore Birkenstocks and had rolled her jeans up past her knees. Jo introduced us. This was Rebecca, and that was her boyfriend, Daniel, on the other side of the yard. They had dropped by for no particular reason except that Jo had wanted us all to meet. I liked Rebecca instantly in the way that I always like people who don't seem to notice my shyness, who act like we've already known each other for years. Rebecca was like that. She sat on my back steps, hugged her knees to her chest, and drank one of the beers from the six-pack that Jo had brought over. Jo opened another and handed it to me.

"It's funny we've never met," Rebecca said, "because I've been to your house a bunch of times."

I didn't ask for explanation. When Jo house-sat for us, she sometimes made dinner for friends. *I was at your house last week*, was a sentence I heard from acquaintances every so often.

"Jo says you're a teacher. Do you like it?" While she spoke, Rebecca gathered her long hair and tied it into a loose bun that instantly came half-undone.

"I love teaching," I said. "Grading is hard. Do you like your work?" I knew from Jo that Rebecca was a nanny. Both of them watched toddlers for long shifts every day, and so they got together often to break up the tedium.

"It's mostly fine. I like kids, but parents can be hard."

Jo rolled her eyes in solidarity.

"I'm trained as an ASL interpreter." Rebecca signed the words as she spoke them, like it was second nature to her. "But it's hard to find that kind of work here." I paused for moment before saying anything. Sign language always transfixed me, like watching murmurations of starlings move together through the sky.

After an hour or so, all three of them rode away on bikes and headed downtown to catch a movie. Kellie found me on the porch and said to me, "Daniel's really cool."

"He is?" I asked, surprised. Though Kellie was friendly to everyone, not many people met her instant approval. It's not that she disliked people, it's that she didn't go about assessing their characters the way I might. When I met a new person, I was always trying to figure out how far I could trust them. Were they worth getting over the awkwardness I'd feel around making small talk? Or would I do better to duck away and fill my hors d'oeuvre plate again? Kellie, on the other hand, moved from person to person with little concern. To hear Kellie say that Daniel was cool meant something.

We saw Daniel and Rebecca one more time a few months later when JoAnn threw a birthday party at her house. We didn't spend much time with them that night, but I saw Daniel through the lens that Kellie had provided. Once I looked at him more closely, it wasn't hard to see what she admired. He was tall and lean with auburn hair and a closely trimmed beard. He was lanky in the same familiar way that my brother was lanky. His voice was smooth. He listened. He seemed serious, although

Jo had told us stories about how funny Daniel was once you knew him well. One night, Jo reported, she and Daniel were sitting on a balcony talking into the wee hours when, without any warning, Daniel stood up and, in one fluid motion, jumped up to the balcony ledge and peed off the side. When surrounded by women, Daniel didn't dominate the conversation or put on any kind of bravado. I agreed with Kellie. I liked that in a guy.

That night at our kitchen table, as we ate chicken and rice and finished the bottle of wine, JoAnn offered to run the idea by Daniel and Rebecca. If they were open to it, we'd arrange a dinner at our house.

Once I had settled into bed, I lay on my side and felt a guarded sense of hope, a small flame below my heart that I carefully tended. If I allowed the flame to grow, I worried that something would go wrong—Daniel would immediately say no, or they'd agree to dinner but stand us up—and I'd be left with only a pile of spent ash. But if I could keep the flame small enough perhaps it would guide us toward something good.

In the end, there wasn't much time for my hope to wane. JoAnn didn't forget or delay. The following afternoon she called me with their answer. Could they come over for dinner next Thursday?

That was six days away. It struck me as a measured time to wait. They weren't overeager, but they were serious.

Kellie and I planned anxiously the Wednesday before. I sat at the kitchen table with a pencil and a notepad, writing down the ingredients we would need. It was a simple list—hamburger buns, meat, a six-pack—one I wouldn't have normally made, but it gave me comfort to write down the things that were in my sphere of control.

"What if they say yes?" I asked her.

"That would be amazing," she said.

"It seems impossible, though."

"Maybe this will be it," she said. She opened her hand, and I gave her the pencil. She used it to doodle on one corner of my list. It was an oval at first, egg-like, that when filled in became a cartoon of a rabbit. "I hope they say yes," Kellie muttered as she drew lines that were whiskers, and I realized that in the two years we'd spent so far looking for a donor and trying to conceive, this was the first moment our hopes had ever been identical.

At ten after six the next evening, Rebecca and Daniel arrived at our door. Side-by-side, they made a sweet pair, both of them in jeans and sandals, which they wriggled out of before stepping into our home. Rebecca cradled a large ceramic bowl of beet salad just above her hip. "I'm sorry we're late," Rebecca explained, handing it to me. "We didn't want to come empty-handed."

"We're just happy that you came at all," Kellie said, taking the bowl from Rebecca.

I nodded at Daniel, and he nodded back. "Welcome," I said.

Once dinner was ready, we spread out across the living room with plates in our laps. Daniel and Rebecca sat on the couch,

Kellie on the chair, and me on the floor, chatting about our jobs and friends we had in common. Now that we were playing it cool, I wondered how we'd ever raise the question. I brooded on this with every bite and found it difficult to chew my food. I told myself that once the plates were in the sink, I'd ask. With every breath, I tried to summon the courage I would need for that moment. But I was still eating when Rebecca spoke up.

"So, we hear you guys want to have a baby."

I looked up from my plate. There is a part of me that would like to pretend that it's a simple thing to ask for sperm. It's not like asking for a kidney. There is no incision, no scalpel, no recovery. But then again, a kidney is straightforward: you give it away so that someone else can live. Doing so makes you noble. You don't have to worry about what that kidney may become someday.

When we asked for sperm, first of all, we were asking for a bodily fluid, which is a little awkward. And, beyond this fleeting awkwardness, how could anyone anticipate what it would feel like to meet (or never meet) a child who carries your family's imprint? What if the child looks just like you? What if you love them? What if you don't?

When I look at these questions head-on, I feel frightened, the way you might when remembering any close call in your life, like when your car skids on black ice and you regain control just before slamming into the guardrail. How easily someone could have been in the neighboring lane. How easily they could have said no.

So when I looked up from my plate that evening, I was checking to see if Daniel was preparing to make a run for it. But, amazingly, he remained on the couch.

"Well, we think that's cool," Rebecca continued. "We'd like to help you with that."

Daniel nodded, like they'd already made a decision.

"You can think about it," I offered.

"It's a lot to consider," Kellie pointed out.

But they were ready to hash out the details. How would it work? They wanted to know. We laid out the two options we'd given Jesse over a year ago. Kellie started by explaining the less intimate option, where Daniel could leave us a stockpile. I jumped in to explain the second option, the DIY option in which we called them every month and arranged a time to pick up a fresh sample.

"We understand if that's just too weird," I apologized. "But for us that would mean fresh sperm, which is better, and fewer logistics."

Rebecca waved a hand through the air. "I think we'd want to do it however it works best for you. The point is to get you pregnant."

Daniel nodded and asked for more details. Was there paperwork to sign? When would we start? Would they get to meet the baby? Would we want them to be involved?

I explained the range of options Kellie and I had considered. If they wanted to take on some kind of aunt and uncle role, we'd be down with that. But at the minimum, we'd want to have a current mailing address.

"Well, of course," Daniel said. "We'd give you as much space as you need."

"But actually, that's not true," Rebecca said. "We'd really want to meet the baby."

I smiled and looked at Kellie. "We'd want that too," I said. I pictured all four of us in a hospital room, passing around a swaddled infant. Then I swallowed, hard. It couldn't be this easy. "Take a week," I told them. "Make sure you mean it."

Rebecca shrugged.

"All right," Daniel said.

At the end of the evening, once the plates had been cleared and we had lingered over dessert, Kellie delivered a warning. "If you do this," she told them, "you guys will wind up pregnant too." I wasn't sure how Kellie had arrived at this conclusion, and yet, it didn't strike me as untrue. I remembered how Jesse's girlfriend had become pregnant in the midst of his talks with us. That was only one example, but still, it seemed like more than a coincidence, that maybe planning for babies filled the air with the idea of them, and maybe the idea of them sometimes made people less careful. Or maybe the intentions I was sending toward my own body were actually traveling in the opposite direction. In any event, Kellie's warning seemed equal parts funny and true.

Rebecca took this all in. "That could happen," she said. "But I sincerely hope you're first."

I dialed Daniel's phone number a week later while pacing my backyard. It was a beautiful day, turning into evening, and the sun was so bright I had to shield my eyes. I was nervous, so I prayed for voice mail, but Daniel answered on the second ring.

"It's Jenn," I said.

"I know," he said. "We haven't changed our minds."

It was a brief conversation that ended with a promise that Kellie or I would call next week when it looked like I was about to ovulate. "We'll be ready," he said. I hung up the phone. My pacing had brought me to the edge of our backyard, and I felt the urge to spread my arms, stand on my tiptoes, and fly over the fence. I was quick to remind myself that the utter faith I felt was foolish. I had no logical reason to believe that home inseminations would yield different results than clinical inseminations. But still, I allowed the flame to burn. I felt free of Dr. Norman, and that freedom felt enough.

16

ACCOUTREMENTS

The modern speculum—the tool shaped like a duckbill and made of plastic or steel—was designed by J. Marion Sims in 1845. You may have heard of him because he's considered the father of modern gynecology. Or, you may have heard of him because he performed dozens of experimental surgeries, all without anesthesia, on enslaved women. He is, today, both famous and infamous: respected for his enduring contributions to obstetrics, and reviled for his methods.

The idea for the speculum came to Sims one morning, after he was called to tend to a white woman who'd been thrown off of a pony and landed on her pelvis. The fall had retroverted her uterus, and Sims manually reset it by entering her digitally and applying great pressure. In doing so, he created a kind of vacuum and "air rushed in and extended the vagina to its fullest capacity." When he removed his hand, the woman let out an immense vaginal fart. "She was exceedingly mortified," Sims reports.[27]

Sims left the incident inspired, realizing that if he could find a way to distend the vagina, he would be able to visually examine his patients. In fact, at that very moment, a young woman named Lucy, who was enslaved, occupied one of his hospital beds with what he thought was an incurable vaginal fistula—a tear in the vaginal wall from a difficult childbirth.

On the way home that morning, Sims bought a pewter spoon.

Soon thereafter, accompanied by two male students, he had Lucy position herself on her hands and knees. The students, one on each side of Lucy, pulled at her butt cheeks (Sims refers to them as "nates") to expose her vagina, into which Sims inserted the bent spoon. Sims writes, "I saw everything, as no man had seen before."[28]

His invention, the duckbill speculum, would allow him to spend the next four years performing experimental surgeries on Lucy and two other women named Betsey and Anarcha, along with several other enslaved women whom he doesn't name in his account. His goal was to perfect a technique for repairing vaginal fistulas, and his many failed experiments resulted in inflammation, agony, and blood poisoning. He casually reports that his final operation on Anarcha was her thirtieth.

In one revealing passage, Sims complains that, while dozens of doctors came to observe and assist his first operations, they eventually tired of watching him fail and, ultimately, he "performed the operations only with the assistance of the patients themselves." Thus enslaved women became, over time, not just the subjects of his experiments, but his assistants. Presumably, they rotated: some recovering from failed surgeries, others enduring those surgeries, and others standing at the doctor's side, handing him the speculum, catheter, sutures.

The speculum was essential to every one of the surgeries he performed. It was the tool that allowed Sims, and the doctors that followed, to examine their patients visually where once they could only palpate.

And the speculum, along with obstetrical forceps and a host of other factors, was an invention that moved the realm of obstetrics, labor, and delivery away from women providers like midwives and into the hands of male doctors.[29] Modern obstetrics as we know it follows a "pathology-oriented" model, one that has routinely used interventions to control the process of delivery rather than simply treating problems as they arise.[30] One example of this is a procedure called the episiotomy, wherein a doctor uses surgical scissors to enlarge the vaginal opening during childbirth. Between 1940 and 1980, under the influence of Dr. Joseph DeLee (the leading obstetrician of his day), episiotomies became standard. The rationale was that the procedure, often combined with the use of forceps, protected both mother and child from injury. Subsequent research, however, has shown that episiotomies are rarely called for, as they often result in undue perineal trauma.[31] Dr. DeLee, like Dr. Sims, was more concerned with influence and innovation than with his true effect on patients.

With his invention, Dr. Sims paved the road for Dr. DeLee, Dr. Norman, and countless others like them—men who make it their life's work to master women's bodies.

These men, in my estimation, relished the control of their position and saw themselves as benevolent helpers doing work they'd been ordained for. And these men, in my estimation, did this work without seeing—truly seeing—their patients. Their perspective was limited to their own ambition and the two-inch view the speculum affords.

To this day, Black women, along with American Indian and Native Alaskan women, are, according to the CDC, "two to three times more likely to die from pregnancy-related causes than white women."[32] There is no convenient rationale for this statistic, no mitigating factor that explains it—it points clearly to a legacy of racism, a systemic dismissal of the pain and symptoms of non-white women. And, while Black women suffer from higher rates of infertility than white women, they are less likely to seek treatment, in part because of a justified suspicion of the medical industry.[33]

The medical realm, so far, was the realm I'd been visiting to conceive a child. The instruments that had been used on me—stirrups, speculum, tenaculum—were not and had never been strictly necessary. That is to say, they were one way, but not the only way, to introduce semen to my body. They were the plastic and metal way, the hospital gown and paper on the table way.

But now that we had changed modes, the accoutrements changed. On the day of our first insemination, Kellie and I sat on our living room floor assembling a small gift for Rebecca and Daniel. Together, we burned a CD with some of our favorite songs, and filled a small ziplock bag with black licorice. It was the kind of offering I would have made for a new best friend in high school, only this time Kellie and I were one couple wooing the friendship of another. We had placed these items in a small, yellow gift bag, not because the offerings themselves warranted wrapping, but because we thought the bag itself might come in handy. Rather than handing over a jar of semen, Daniel could place that jar inside the gift bag. In this way, we might preserve a sense of boundary between us. The bag, like magic, would transform fluid in the jar from his to ours.

Kellie tucked me into our bed before she left for Rebecca and Daniel's, and I waited for her beneath the covers, naked and worried. Outside, a September wind blew through the branches of our fir tree. They waved back and forth like arms. I fixed my eyes on those branches—the smooth gray bark and the pale green needles—and I tried to calm my body down. But my body wouldn't take direction. My heart sped, and my mind turned over on itself. I kept imagining a scenario where Kellie would knock on their door and wait for an answer but no one would come. She'd knock again and wait some more, and finally

Rebecca would appear. She'd open the door just enough to stick out her head and whisper the news that this just wasn't going to work.

This seemed likely to me: that the body might resist performing on command, that there might be no bigger turnoff in the world than a phone call demanding an ejaculation. It would be reasonable, I thought, to decide in that moment of truth, half-naked in the bathroom, that this whole idea was a big mistake. I counted the minutes and expected Kellie to come home empty-handed. With every minute that passed, this scenario seemed more and more inevitable. I watched the clock and calculated: fifteen minutes to drive across town, fifteen minutes to return. How long would the exchange take? I wondered. Would they stand in the doorway and chat for a while? Would she simply take the jar and leave?

Kellie returned without the yellow bag. I sat up in bed to crane my neck and see if she was empty-handed.

"What happened?" I asked, the moment she entered the room. Kellie placed an object on my bedside table. It was a brown wool pouch with a jar inside. Kellie worked to untie the knot.

"They didn't need our bag," Kellie said. "They had one already." As Kellie opened the jar and prepared the syringe, I inspected the pouch. I was struck by how nest-like it was. The weave was loose and the wool was scraggled; it bunched in places, and thread poked out here and there. That pouch, more than anything, signaled that we had arrived on new terrain.

Sperm no longer came in a tiny vial; it came in a canning jar, like one of the many that lined the shelves in my pantry. Sperm was no longer thawed, spun, and placed under a microscope—instead it was kept warm against my partner's belly as she transported it from one side of town to another.

There were no stirrups, no tenaculums, no instruments of torture. There was no Dr. Norman, just Kellie, who now gave the syringe her full concentration as she pulled on the plunger. "Wow," she commented as the reservoir filled. "We can fill more than one of these."

I had thought the three syringes on the table were overkill, just a precaution or a superstition. When we inseminated at the clinic, the full sample always seemed to fit inside a single 5 ml syringe. But Kellie finished filling the first, and then she went on to fill the second and part of the third. (I would later learn that specimens purchased from sperm banks are only a fraction of the total ejaculate. The typical single donation is divided into as many as twenty straws or vials.)

I liked having Kellie as my doctor. She was kinder than Dr. Norman—and much cuter. As she picked up the full syringe, I pulled down the covers and bent my knees. She held up my legs with one arm and did her job gently, carefully, seriously, and when she was done, she took off her shoes and her pants and got under the covers.

We didn't have much time to linger. That morning, when Kellie called to arrange a pickup time, she had also invited

Daniel and Rebecca to come by for dinner afterward. When they said yes, we had invited Jo too. Our intention had been to cultivate friendship, to try and keep things reciprocal somehow, but I felt awkward about it now—why hadn't we thought to schedule it for later in the week? It seemed like a strange situation to carry on casual conversation with someone whose semen you had just injected inside of you, whose sperm might be at that very moment swimming toward your egg.

Kellie looked at the clock. "Stay here as long as you can," she said. "I'll go pick up the pizza."

With Kellie gone from the bed again, I propped up my torso with a pillow. I lifted my legs and pointed my toes toward the ceiling. I looked again at the branches outside. The wind had settled.

When I finally got up from the bed, I pulled on my jeans and brought the jar to the kitchen with me. I turned it around in my hand. I wasn't sure what I was supposed to do with it. Should I clean it with a regular sponge? Once it was clean, what then? Would we shelve it with the canning jars, or should I mark it with tape and a Sharpie? Would it now become our official sperm jar? I wasn't sure, so I filled it with warm water, noted how the trace of semen turned the water cloudy, and left it there to soak.

JoAnn arrived with a bottle of wine just moments before Daniel and Rebecca. I was busy using the bathroom as JoAnn uncorked the bottle and served herself, so I didn't notice what glass she had chosen until I turned around to see her sitting at the kitchen table, drinking wine from a little round jar. I looked at her, and then I looked in the sink. The sperm jar was gone. JoAnn took a sip. I looked at Daniel and Rebecca, and then JoAnn again, waiting to see if anyone would figure it out.

I knew it would be wrong to say nothing. I was pretty sure she hadn't washed it, or at she least hadn't washed it in the way that you would if you were planning to drink from a container that had recently been used to inseminate your friend.

But I didn't know how to say it, right there in front of Daniel, without everyone dying of embarrassment. I imagined all of our faces flushing red, the rest of the evening continuing in strained silence. Finally, I just blurted it out.

"Jo," I said gently, "I am so sorry, but I can't let you drink out of that jar."

Jo looked down at her wine and then back at me. She didn't understand. I looked to Daniel, hoping he might help me. He coughed into his hand.

"Oh!" she said finally, and we all burst out in laughter. "Oh shit."

Daniel reached an arm in her direction. "Just give it to me," he said. "No big deal for me to drink it."

Jo handed him the jar and stood up to start a new glass for herself. Kellie's truck pulled into the driveway. I fetched three more glasses, filled them for Rebecca and Kellie, and poured myself a quarter glass of wine for toasting. Together, we drank.

17
LAST-DITCH EFFORTS

With Daniel and Rebecca on our side, failure changed for me.
When my period arrived that month and the month after that, I
felt a cleaner sense of disappointment. I wanted to be pregnant,
and I wasn't. That was all. I no longer felt like the world was
against me.

Still, I felt the need to make every month count. In my mind,
the timer ticked on—it wasn't just my own biological clock I was
tracking, but Rebecca and Daniel's patience. I wondered how
many months they would last before the novelty of helping us
wore off. It seemed impossible to me that they could continue
indefinitely without being infected by my own disappointment.
If I knew anything, it was this: perpetual failure is a drag.

Adding to my fear was the fact that their lives had recently
become more complicated. Daniel had taken a job in Seattle,
and they had found a rental there. Rebecca still worked in
Olympia, where Daniel owned a house, so they were temporarily

straddling life between two cities sixty miles apart. I worried that we might have already become one more obligation in their too-busy lives.

"They're not sick of us yet," Kellie reassured me one evening as we drove to Seattle. "It's only our third month." It was the middle of the workweek, I was due to ovulate, and so we were on our way to their new home. We had waited for traffic to clear, the sun had gone down, and now we sped along the interstate through long dark stretches, through bright industrial zones, and then finally into Daniel and Rebecca's new neighborhood. As we pulled into their driveway, Rebecca appeared in the doorway, her dog already on a leash. She squinted at our headlights and waved, a slicker pulled over her head.

"We're ready for you," Rebecca said, motioning us to come in. Daniel was putting his jacket on behind her, completing his Pacific Northwest winter uniform of jeans, flannel, and rain gear.

"The donation's in the bathroom," Daniel told us. "Make yourselves at home."

"You're welcome to our bed," Rebecca added. "How long do you need? An hour?"

"Thirty minutes tops," I said. The rain had been stopping and starting all day, and I didn't like the idea of sending them out in the weather. "You don't have to leave," I added.

"We'd be walking the dog anyways," Rebecca reassured me.

As we slipped inside, Daniel ushered us toward the bathroom. Their new apartment was a converted shed—a small ground floor with a bathroom and kitchenette, and a wood ladder that led to a loft. It would have been impossible to guess you were in Seattle just by looking around; their place looked more like a forest cabin with its wood-paneled walls, sleeping loft, and the single window over the kitchen sink.

The jar of semen sat in its wool bag in a box by a space heater, which had been set to low. Neither Kellie nor I wanted to take over Daniel and Rebecca's bed, so I lay on the bath mat next to their shower and took off my pants. The bathroom floor was cold.

Once Kellie had finished her part of the job, she returned to the car to grab the magazine she'd brought. Alone on the floor in the bathroom, my mind began to wander.

In the last couple of weeks, I'd been rethinking my stance on doctors. Dr. Norman had failed me—I felt sure of that—and I had felt a certain glee at leaving him behind, but I kept circling around to the truth of things: I was a single body, a pair of lungs, a set of ribs, a single heart. There was no second being inside of me, no alternate heartbeat, no someday-baby. My body was alone. I wanted to believe it was possible that I could get pregnant without any further intervention, that Rebecca and Daniel's generosity would be enough to right whatever was broken in me. I wanted to believe that, but I didn't.

So far all our babymaking expenses had come out of pocket. But a few days earlier, because it was open enrollment time at Kellie's workplace, Kellie came home with a brochure that outlined her health insurance benefits. I was insured through my own workplace and had never compared our plans before, but this time I studied the list of covered conditions carefully and discovered that her plan offered something rare: fertility diagnostics. Kellie's plan would not pay for inseminations, nor would they shell out tens of thousands of dollars for in vitro fertilization, but they would pay for the blood tests, ultrasounds, and laparoscopies that might help identify the problem. And since we had now been trying to conceive for over a year, someone out there—someone other than Dr. Norman—might take me seriously. If I signed up this month, my coverage would begin on January 1. That was two months away.

As I lay now on the bath mat, naked below the waist, legs balanced above my head, yoga-style, I stared at the shower curtain, which was covered in giant multicolored polka dots. I traced the rows with my eyes. I prayed, as I always prayed, that this time would work. I prayed also that, if it didn't, we would soon find some kind of answer. I gathered all my energy and hoped.

When Rebecca and Daniel returned, all four of us loaded into their station wagon in search of a late dinner. It was raining now in earnest; the windshield wipers hummed, and as we moved through the dark, me in the back seat with Kellie, I felt cocooned. Daniel drove, and Rebecca shifted her body to talk to us over the seat.

"How are you guys feeling?" she asked. "Is this the month?"

Her enthusiasm touched me, but I needed her to ration

her hope. "I don't know," I said. "This whole thing could take a while." I launched into an explanation of my plan, probably presenting more detail than they were ready for. "We don't want to keep you on the hook forever."

We pulled up at a stop sign, and Daniel turned his head for a moment, and then continued driving. "It's all right," he said, his voice gravelly and calm. "We're trying to make a human being." His voice turned to wonder when he said it—*a human being.* Rebecca put a hand over his hand. I thought once more of the end goal: a warm living body that was separate from my own. All those cells and veins and neural pathways. All that skin and sinew and bone. No wonder it was taking a while. No wonder it took time, intention, patience. As we parked in front and left the car, my body, which had become a cage of worry, loosened ever so slightly.

I visited the fertility clinic in Tacoma on January 4, two days before I was scheduled to ovulate, and four days before my thirty-first birthday.

The office in Tacoma fit the picture I originally had of what a fertility office should look like. It looked like money. It had dark leather couches, frosted glass doors, and brand-new carpets with geometric patterns. I waited for only five minutes before the doctor came out, shook my hand, and beckoned me into her office. I imagined that today she'd simply take down my history and send back to the reception desk with instructions to schedule a future exam. I didn't imagine that I would leave that day any closer to solving my body's mystery.

Dr. Katz was shorter than I was. She was a white woman about twenty years my senior, who wore small silver earrings and pink lipstick. When I shook her hand, it was soft and dry. She didn't blink when I revealed that I was a lesbian, but she was concerned about our donor situation.

"Do you have a lawyer?" she asked me.

"Not yet," I admitted. I wasn't worried that Daniel or Rebecca would ever try to seek custody, but I understood that to an outsider our situation sounded like a disaster waiting to happen.

"Do me a favor and get one," she said.

Once Dr. Katz had filled in all of the blanks, she surprised me by looking up from her desk.

"So you're close to ovulation?" she asked.

"Yes."

"Well, this is really good timing." She looked up at her clock and then back at me. "I'd like to get you under the ultrasound. Is that okay?"

Never in my life would I have ever imagined that the phrase "get you under the ultrasound" would make my heart soar with gratitude, but it did. "Yes," I said. "Yes, I'm fine with that."

Moments later, I was in a hospital gown in a bright exam room down the hall from her office. Dr. Katz pulled a glove over her right hand and spread some prewarmed lube across my belly. She looked over at the screen, which was covered in shades of black, white, and gray. She studied the vague shapes my organs made. She pointed to the projection of my ovaries. "I'm not seeing as many ripe follicles as I'd like to." She continued to move the probe across my belly. "But more importantly," she went on, "I'm seeing texture on your uterus that looks like endometriosis."

I knew a little about endometriosis, from a roommate I'd had years ago who had spent several days of every month doubled up in pain. She would lie in her bed with a jar of herbal tea and emerge into the kitchen every so often, stooped and bleary-eyed. She had told me that her periods were excruciating because her womb was covered in scar tissue. "Why?" I had asked. "No reason," she told me, then added, "My body is reactive."

My periods weren't excruciating. They were painful, that was all. But I had wondered sometimes about endometriosis, because I knew my body was reactive too. I had asthma and eczema, conditions that meant that in the interest of protecting me, my body caused itself damage. In reaction to allergens, my skin swelled and wept, then cracked and bled. When I walked through cold winter air, my bronchi narrowed and went into spasm. I could imagine my uterus doing a similar thing, growing layers of scar tissue to compensate for some perceived wound.

Dr. Katz explained now that scar tissue often prevented a zygote from implanting. "So it's possible that there's no problem with the sperm reaching your eggs," she said. "But once that zygote travels down the tube, it's got nowhere to land."

She went on to lay out the procedure that she was likely to prescribe. They would make a small incision in my belly and send a laparoscope inside of me to remove the extra tissue. Once I healed, my uterus would be clear and hospitable. If all went well, I would conceive.

She couldn't do this right away, though. She wanted me to come back next month for another diagnostic. In this test, they would send blue dye through my cervix. The dye would spread through my womb, like food coloring in water, and they would verify that my fallopian tubes were clear, that my uterus was truly the problem.

"So is it worth it to try this month?" I asked her.

"Definitely try," she instructed. "It won't hurt anything."

I left her office full of joy and fury. Joy because someone had finally offered me an answer. Fury because all it had taken was one appointment, one ultrasound, one half of one hour; because my problem might have easily been solved a year ago when I first started asking questions. Dr. Norman, I was certain, had an ultrasound on-site. He billed himself as a fertility specialist. Had it never occurred to him to take a look at what was going on? Did straight women typically get an ultrasound before proceeding to insemination or IVF? Was this one more example of how lesbians could easily fall through the cracks after being diagnosed with Male Factor Infertility?

And what about Dr. Tran, the obstetrician I'd sought out after my initial failed attempts? I had described to her in detail my feeling that I was conceiving each month but then bleeding on time, and she had sent me away with a progesterone prescription, telling me there was nothing else she could do. But the symptoms I described to her aligned with Dr. Katz's description of endometriosis. It struck me that if Dr. Tran hadn't shooed me away—if she had listened and believed me—she might have helped me find the problem many months ago.

Dr. Katz was the kind of doctor that I'd long ago assumed I'd encounter when we first began planning for a child: she was professional, clinical, helpful, and unfazed by my orientation. If my having a same-sex partner made me an unusual client in her practice, she didn't let me know it.

And yet, if we had seen her on day one, would she have proceeded any differently than Dr. Norman had? Would she have asked for tests after a several rounds of failures? Or would she have simply put us on the same track that Dr. Norman had—six inseminations and then on to in vitro—and failed to investigate further?

I walked into Dr. Katz's office as a woman who had tried and failed to conceive for over a year. In other words, I walked into her office as someone who, in that particular way, resembled her typical straight patients, and perhaps this is the reason she was able to so easily diagnose me, to find in mere minutes the answer I'd spent two years pursuing. I had stepped into the right place at the right time to bypass the ways in which it was not designed for me.

———————

It was late on a Sunday morning, three days after my appointment, when Daniel called. "Are we still doing this?" he asked. I was due to ovulate at any moment, and he was cleaning his Olympia house, preparing to leave it for the last time. Rebecca had already left for Seattle, her station wagon packed with their remaining boxes. She had left her job and now she'd be living in Seattle full time too. Daniel was calling now to see if bringing us sperm was one more item he needed to add to his to-do list.

"Yeah," I said, feeling guilty. "I still want to."

Daniel promised to drop by with a jar on his way out of town, though he couldn't name a time.

"That's okay," I said. "I'll just be home."

It seemed that no one besides me had too much hope for this month. After my appointment with Dr. Katz, I had called Rebecca from my cell phone in my driveway—it was an excuse to stay in my car a few minutes longer before walking through the rain to go inside. Rebecca had answered on the first ring. "How'd it go?" she said, as if she'd been waiting for my call.

I described the ultrasound, the grainy image of my scar-covered uterus, my imminent surgery.

"So that's it, you think?" she asked. "We'll just take a break, they'll fix you up, and we'll be pregnant before you know it?"

I loved it that Rebecca said "we."

It struck me now that everyone—Daniel, Rebecca, Kellie—had moved their hope into the future. This time would be a last-ditch effort, pretty much dispensable. But I didn't see it that way. A friend had once described to me her experience getting a hysterosalpingogram, the procedure that Dr. Katz had suggested I try next month. She described watching the blue dye spread through her fallopian tubes on the fluoroscope. She said the images were beautiful, and also that it was the worst pain she'd ever felt in her life. I knew that a successful conception this month was a long shot, but I also knew that if I could avoid that procedure and a subsequent surgery, I wanted to.

Kellie was cleaning gutters when Daniel finally showed up. I intercepted him before he had a chance to knock, and he handed me a jar wrapped inside a T-shirt. I took it. The driver's side door was open and the car was running. It was raining again. "Drive safe!" I hollered as he bolted back down the steps. Daniel waved to Kellie on the roof before driving off.

I stood just inside the doorway with the jar. If I hollered for Kellie, I'd need to wait for her to climb down the ladder, to remove her boots and the layers of muddy clothes she was wearing for the job. The whole endeavor might take nearly ten minutes, and as each minute passed we'd lose more and more sperm.

I decided to inseminate myself, though I felt strangely alone as I did it. As I filled the syringe, lay down on the bed, parted my legs, found the tilt of my opening, and pressed the plunger into the reservoir, I could feel my ghost self hover above my real self, watching. Alone, alone, alone.

Moments later the front door opened, and I could hear Kellie pull off her boots and unzip her layers. She entered the bedroom. "Shit," she said. "Did you do my job?"

I nodded. My sadness about being alone instantly evaporated. She had arrived and I hadn't had to ask.

"Oh well," she said as she climbed in next to me, her feet, her hands, and her face cold from being on the roof. I held her hands between my hands, pressed my feet against her feet. We lay there together, my skin warming hers, the sky outside a January gray, the rain falling on drenched earth.

I was still two days away from turning thirty-one. In four days I would see a massage therapist who would ask me what conditions I was hoping to treat. I would look down at the floor beneath the wheels of her table and confess that I'd been trying for two years to get pregnant. "Mmm," she would say. It was a noise of understanding. "It took me four years to get pregnant." Later she would cup her hands around my heels and gently pull. She would cradle the base of my skull and send me away feeling just a little longer, a little stretched, a little healed. "Seek as much pleasure as you can," was her advice to me.

Strangely, this was the resolution I'd already come to over the last month. In fact, this was why I had sought her in the first place. No more acupuncture, no more long drives to Seattle, no more lying on the table with pins in my ears and ankles wondering when Dr. Xiao would release me. As I braced myself for another year of trying and waiting, waiting and trying, I decided I would endure by letting go of things I didn't want to do.

Pleasure would be my new medicine. I would sleep late whenever I could, pull my covers close to me and look out the window. I would tear pieces from a fresh baguette and fold them around tranches of cold butter. I would go on long runs, take long showers, and neglect my to-do list whenever I could.

———————

On the day my period was due, less than two weeks after my birthday, I woke up in a new bed, on an island in British Columbia. The birds were chirping so loudly and ecstatically that they'd woken me. I looked out the window and couldn't see a single one—just a stand of red alders—but they were undeniably there.

We were on Gabriola Island because Kellie had received a call earlier in the week. Over the summer, she had inquired about a three-month intensive program at the Island School of Building Arts. It was a dream she'd kept secret for a while—a desire to build cabins out of whole logs and hearths out of river rock—but once she finally contacted them, she learned the program was already full. She was number eighteen on a wait list. We hadn't planned on her getting in. But it was January now, the program started in three months, and suddenly a spot had opened up. If Kellie took it, she'd have to leave her steady job.

Kellie tried to convince me that it was a foolish risk. She was forty-three and female. "The only people leaving that program with a job are the men in their twenties," she said.

"You don't know that," I said. I wanted her to go. Her job seemed to dim her. She came home looking weary, not because the work was too hard, but because it wasn't hard enough. Besides, I tried to convince her, the timing was good. Unless I were pregnant right now, it would be at least three months before we were trying again, a year or more before we'd have a newborn. If Kellie wanted to take off for an island, to change jobs or careers, this was the final window.

And so we had rented a B and B room with heated floors and a queen-size bed. In my overnight bag, I had packed a pregnancy test. I told myself there was a practical reason for this. As we visited the school and weighed Kellie's options, it would be good to know if I was, at that moment, carrying a child. But the truer reason was this: I felt a certain lightness when I pictured the freshly made bed and the bathroom that would be immaculate, clean from every association that my own bathroom carried.

When I got out of bed that morning, I said nothing to Kellie as I unpacked the pregnancy test from my toiletry bag, brought it to the bathroom, and peed. The bathroom floors were heated too, the walls a mosaic of small, colored tiles. I didn't watch the test; I didn't wait for the result to reveal itself before my very eyes. Instead, I put on a show for whatever gods might be watching, pretending I had arrived at some kind of patience. I left the bathroom, laid out my clothes for the day on the bed, and got ready for the shower. I had only my underwear on when I returned to the bathroom and picked up the test. I looked.

The result was clear.

Through the open door, I could see Kellie over her duffel bag, dressing for the day, but I stood silent for a moment, stunned. I wasn't sure what to say.

"Hey, want to see something?" I called out finally, my voice cracking.

Kellie appeared in the doorway. "What?" she asked.

"I took a test," I told her. I handed her the plastic stick.

She picked it up and examined the window.

"You see two lines, right?"

"Yeah," she said. "But one of them is faint."

This was true, but I knew by heart the instructions on the box. "It's not supposed to matter." I placed the test back on top of the toilet, as if the answer might grow even more definitive if it rested there another minute.

Kellie stepped forward to pull me against her. Her wool sweater scratched against my bare skin. "That's something, huh?" she said.

I nodded. "We'll see."

That day, as we toured the grounds of the Island School, as I stepped over piles of sawdust and examined half-built homes and stacks of peeled logs, I tried to tune in to whatever was growing inside of me. If it was truly there, it was a tiny thing, smaller than a seed. I sent it good thoughts; I willed it to thrive.

On our drive back to our room along the island's one arterial road, we passed fields of sheep, old farmhouses, views of the Georgia Strait.

"Do you think this could be it?" I asked Kellie.

"You tell me," she said. She kept one hand on the wheel and reached for me with the other. "Is this it?"

"Fifty-fifty chance," I said. I couldn't help but imagine my period arriving in the next day or two. But in my mind I negotiated with that number; I asked it to climb up to seventy, eighty, ninety.

Four days later, Kellie and I sat on the couch in the evening. She had just dialed Daniel, and the line was ringing.

My period still hadn't arrived. Dr. Katz's office had directed me to take a blood test, and earlier that day, a nurse had called with the results. She told me my levels looked strong, and I asked if I should worry about Dr. Katz's proposed diagnosis. "No," she said. "Conception is the hard part. No cure for endometriosis like a healthy pregnancy."

Daniel picked up. "We've got news for you," Kellie said, and then she handed me the phone.

"What's up?" Daniel asked, and I was struck by how unsuspecting he sounded.

"So…" I stalled for a moment. "I'm pregnant."

"No way!" he shouted, his voice cracking with genuine surprise. "Damn," he said. "Wow."

"I know."

"Thank god for last-ditch efforts, right?"

I handed the phone to Kellie and rested my feet in her lap. Daniel knew now, and soon Rebecca would too. I knew that the etiquette of pregnancy meant that, out in the world, I'd have to keep my news a secret. It gave me joy to have a reason to break the silence this way, to have this new family we were making extend beyond ourselves.

18

I WORRY

Worry became my prayer, my way of holding vigil. If I held this baby in my mind during every waking moment, perhaps it wouldn't leave me. At this point, after two years of trying, I found it hard to believe that my body wouldn't bleed, that I wouldn't flush away this growing thing. Flushing was my body's habit; it knew no other way, and so I spoke to my body constantly, instructing it—pleading with it. I closed my eyes and imagined nine months without bleeding. How could such magic be possible?

I kept reminding myself of the nurse on the phone who had told me I had no reason to worry. But I had every reason to worry. My body had failed me over and over.

I could not use the bathroom without fearing that I'd find a bloodstain on my underwear, or that I'd leave a drop of red behind to spread in the toilet water, or that when I wiped I'd see a trace of pink. I could imagine these details so easily. To ward off my fear, I developed an elaborate set of rituals.

At work, I could only use the first-floor bathroom, first stall on the left. It was a stall I'd rarely used before I conceived. I had never bled in that particular toilet, never changed a sanitary napkin there, and so I trusted that stall to keep me safe.

Wherever I went, I held my breath as I pulled down my pants. I stretched the crotch of my underwear between my two fingers and inspected the fabric for anything resembling blood. I learned to carefully wad the toilet paper before I wiped, otherwise the pink of my finger might show through a single ply and startle me. It would take me minutes for my heart rate to recover from the sight of what I thought was blood.

Because so far I had no pregnancy symptoms, the worrying was all I had, the only difference between pregnant me and me alone. If I didn't worry, if I didn't spend all of my mental energy on protecting this thing that was growing, then how could I be sure it was there?

By week six, my nausea competed with my worry. It began on Super Bowl Sunday, when my brother came over to our house with a giant bowl of seven-layer bean dip and a bag of tortilla chips. He had recently moved to Olympia to spend a year finishing college. The house he rented was one block away from me.

I still always referred to Nick as my little brother. He had no recollection of me cradling him and changing his diapers, but those moments would always inform who he was to me. And Super Bowl Sunday was typical of the kind of time we'd spend together: I didn't care about football, but I liked any excuse to share space with Nick.

I scooped dip onto the plate and began to eat as Nick and Kellie watched the game. I hadn't eaten since breakfast, and my stomach was raging, but something made me slow down. There was something about the squish of the guacamole, the smoothness of the sour cream, the density of the cold beans that made me gag. I kept going though; it tasted good. As I dipped my chips, I marveled at how odd it was to enjoy something and be repulsed by it at the same time.

Within two weeks, there was nothing in the world I wanted to eat. I didn't vomit, but every smell made me gag. One morning I put a waffle in the toaster because it seemed like the most innocuous food I could think of. As it thawed and heated, the smell spread through the kitchen with an intensity I'd never before noticed. Flour and buttermilk were smells I would have once considered neutral. Now, I was surprised by my own disgust. A waffle. I couldn't handle the smell of a waffle.

I'd expected the nausea, but nothing had prepared me for the fatigue. When I read about the symptoms of pregnancy, I had interpreted the word fatigue to mean the state of being sleepy, tired, worn out. I had felt those things before. I thought I knew fatigue. I imagined that maybe I'd go to bed early some nights or that I'd want an occasional nap.

Week seven taught me that I had no idea what fatigue really was. I didn't feel like I would have felt after not sleeping well for a few nights in a row. I didn't feel like I had hiked up a mountain or taken a red-eye flight across the country. Instead, I felt like a strong wave had knocked me underwater and into the sand. I could struggle to get up, only to be knocked down again by the next oncoming wave. I didn't crave sleep, and it didn't restore me. I climbed into bed whenever I could, not because a nap sounded nice but because gravity itself was strenuous.

I worried that, to Kellie, it would appear that I was acting. There was little evidence for my new condition: no vomiting, no fever, no hacking cough that would prove how sick I felt. I tried to explain it to her one morning. It was a Saturday, and she had driven us to a nearby harbor to watch the seals. I stood on the shore, a February wind whipping my hair; I held the binoculars to my eyes to watch the seals belly up to the docks. The sky was clear. The sun was bright. It hurt my eyes. It tired me. I lasted less than ten minutes before asking Kellie how long she wanted to stay.

"I know it seems weird," I told her as she drove us home. I leaned my head against the window and pressed my forehead to the glass. "I can't even describe it. I've never been so tired in my life."

Kellie shrugged. She dropped me off at home and left to continue with her day. I slept for a full two hours, a thin and drooling sleep. Every twenty minutes I woke up, looked at the clock, and commanded my body to move, but then the weight of my head pulled me back to my pillow.

I could tell I was scaring Kellie a little. Later, when I was finally awake, she came home to find me sitting with a cup of green tea, trying to drink it sip by tiny sip, trying to ignore its awful bitter taste, hoping the small dose of caffeine might give me energy.

Instead of dinner now, I made oatmeal and let Kellie fend for herself. Left to her own devices, Kellie had always been happy to eat the same thing every night. She heated a plain tortilla in the toaster oven until it was nearly burned, sliced some cheddar cheese, and then covered the whole thing with sriracha. She didn't care that I'd stopped cooking. She cared that I was disappearing. "I'm losing you," she said. "That baby's already taking everything you've got."

She was kind of kidding, kind of not. I couldn't laugh; I couldn't answer. I could only take another sip of bitter tea and stare out the window, hoping to feel something different soon.

Kellie worried about leaving me behind. In less than a month, she would leave for the Island School as I entered my second trimester. For three months, she wouldn't come home, though I would visit her on alternate weekends.

"What are you going to do if you still feel like this?" she asked me.

"I won't," I promised. "Everyone says I'll feel better."

"It's like magic," Victoria had told me. "One morning you wake up and feel like yourself again." I found it hard to believe her. The thing I didn't tell Kellie was that, with the way I was feeling right now, I didn't need her at all. The illness of pregnancy was, for me, a very solitary thing. Kellie couldn't sleep on my behalf or show up at work in my place. She couldn't cook for me because there was nothing I wanted to eat. In bed at night, she couldn't even touch me. The nausea made me so constantly seasick that any touch made me want to crawl out of my skin.

Kellie departed in her diesel truck on a Sunday morning in March. She had her tools packed and organized, her cold-weather clothes in two duffel bags. Since Kellie had been the last student to register, she'd been assigned to the only short-term rental left: a half-finished shack in a family's backyard. Kellie would call me to report that her shack was full of spiders and that the frogs inhabiting the adjacent marsh were so loud that they kept her up all night. Monday morning she would put on her bright orange rain gear over her work clothes and drive through a downpour to move logs and cut laps with a dozen men.

By the time Kellie left, it was clear that the magic of the second trimester was on its way. Food still repulsed me to some degree, but I could eat without crying. My fatigue had dwindled until it felt like everyday tired and not soul-crushing tired. The thought of having our house to myself for the next three months did not frighten me, except for one small concern. If my pregnancy ended, or if anything went wrong, I would not want to be there alone.

19

THIS IS A TEST

When my phone rang on a Monday morning and the voice on the other end identified herself as Samantha from Prenatal Diagnosis, I assumed that she was calling with good news.

I had opted into a series of tests called Integrated Prenatal Screening—a combination of one ultrasound and two blood draws meant to identify increased risk for genetic conditions and neural tube defects. The result of the combined tests would not be a definitive answer, but rather, a statistical likelihood. Because I was thirty-one, my statistical chance of carrying a baby with Down syndrome was about one in a thousand; for Trisomy 18 it was one in eight thousand. Those were the general statistics, available to anyone on the internet. But this test would look for specific hormones in my own blood and somehow, through a process that was mysterious to me, assess if my risk was greater than average. Victoria, for instance, reported that she had taken the test and they had told her that there was a one-in-four-thousand chance her baby had Down syndrome.

I had taken the test because I had wanted the reassurance of numbers. I knew that 5 percent of people who took the test screened positive, and that they were the ones who would go on to make hard decisions. Would they simply live with the uncertainty and wait until the child revealed everything at birth? Would they get an amniocentesis? If the amnio revealed an abnormality, would they terminate? I didn't expect that I would have to answer these questions.

I expected Samantha now to offer me a ratio like one-in-nine-hundred or one-in-twelve-thousand, some fraction of a percentage, a risk so small I could pinch it between my fingers. I was eager to receive the good news.

Also, I was eager to be done with Samantha, my assigned genetic counselor. I had met her once before, when she had summoned me from the waiting room. I was there for my ultrasound and consultation—the first part of my screening process—and I had instructed Kellie to stay in Olympia that day and go to work as normal. I didn't want Kellie there. I was anxious about the appointment and wouldn't have minded having her company, but the price for that would be too high. Our early experiences at Dr. Norman's clinic had trained me. I didn't want to have to explain who Kellie was, or catch sideways glances in the waiting room, or even to have to wonder about what other people might be thinking. It was easier to go it alone.

But Kellie was anxious too, and so she kept calling me for updates. "You learn anything?" she asked me, just one minute after my appointment was scheduled to start.

"I'm still in the waiting room," I told her. This was the moment that Samantha, a young white woman with a tight ponytail, appeared at the end of the corridor and called my name. "I gotta go," I told Kellie before flipping my phone shut and stuffing it in my coat pocket.

Samantha introduced herself, and I followed behind her as she led the way to her office. She wore a lab coat with a pencil skirt, gray stockings, and one-inch heels. She had a glossy smile. "Was that your husband on the phone?" she asked as she pointed me to a seat in the corner of her office.

"My partner," I told her. I was glad to get that out of the way.

"Great!" she said. She settled into her own chair with a clipboard and a ballpoint pen. "I'll be spending some time with you today. I need to take down your family's medical history."

As I answered her questions, I wondered how she would address the other half of my baby's genetic background.

Samantha turned a page on her clipboard. "So, your partner," she began, "does he have any current medical problems?"

"Um, my partner is a woman," I told her. "We used sperm from a donor."

Samantha looked up from her clipboard. Her face had turned pink; I could see the heat spreading from her cheeks to the tips of her ears. "Oh my gosh," she said. "I'm so sorry." She returned her gaze to the clipboard and fumbled with her papers, looking through them as if she had lost something between the pages. "Do we have to start all over now? I mean, was it even your egg?" She seemed not just flustered, but distressed.

"It's my egg," I said. I wanted her to calm down. I kept my body still, my voice even, hoping that her reaction would just crash over me like a wave and subside.

But as I sat still, my mind spun questions. This woman worked every day with pregnant women. This was Seattle, one of the most progressive cities in the country. Did she think that lesbians didn't ovulate? In her graduate program, did they never discuss alternative families? Or was she absent that day? Even if she'd never met a lesbian before, hadn't some of her clients conceived with donor sperm or eggs? I struggled to understand how she was so thoroughly unprepared for this moment.

Samantha continued to riffle through the papers on her clipboard, absolutely perplexed. "I'm sorry," she said again.

"Look," I said. "Our donor is a friend. Why don't you just ask me your questions and I'll do my best to answer them."

"Okay," she agreed. Her voice trembled a bit as she ran through her list. She didn't make eye contact with me again. "I'm so sorry," she said.

"It's fine," I said. It was the third time she had said she was sorry, and each time she said it, the words carried a double meaning for me. She was sorry she'd made an assumption, but also she was sorry for me, the way she would be sorry if I had told her I had a disease.

On the phone now in my quiet house, I waited for Samantha to keep talking, to offer the results of the blood test. I had moved to the spot where my older dog was sleeping on his side; I laid my hand on the rise of his chest. His fur was soft there, and white. He rolled to his back and lifted his paws to accommodate my touch.

"I have some hard news," she said.

"Oh." I moved my hand down to my dog's lower belly and rested it there. My dog pushed my hand with his paw, urging me to keep scratching. "Okay."

Samantha told me that she had the results from my blood work in front of her. She reminded me that the typical risk for a woman my age to carry a child with Down syndrome was somewhere around one in a thousand. "Your result shows an increased risk. Your odds are one in sixty."

"Oh." I covered my throat with my hand. My dog pawed at me again, but I didn't pet him. "What's my next step?" I asked, but I already knew the answer. If I wanted to know for sure, I would need to get an amniocentesis, where a doctor would press a long needle through layers of abdominal flesh and muscle all the way through to the baby's amniotic sac. The needle would take a sample of amniotic fluid. Though the results would be definitive—a yes or a no instead of a one-in-sixty chance— there was a small possibility that the sac would rupture, that I would leak all of my amniotic fluid, that the baby I was carrying would die.

This was my choice now: I'd get an amniocentesis, or I'd live with the mystery for another five months. A thread of panic ran from my stomach to my throat.

"Well, what would you do if your baby had Down syndrome?" Samantha asked me. Her tone was casual, almost cheery. "Would you terminate?"

I stammered. "I, um, I don't know. I think I'd want that information."

I'd read once about a young mother who carried a pregnancy to term even though her baby was destined to live no longer than a week. She carried the baby, labored with the baby, she held him and nursed him for the forty-eight hours he lived, and then she said goodbye. I read about her with tears streaming down my cheeks, in awe of the courage it takes to love something that you know you will lose. For the first time, it had occurred to me that unconditional love might mean seeing your baby through from beginning to end, no matter what their genetic code carried.

But although this woman's choice struck me as brave, I didn't think I would choose this. If I learned that I was carrying a baby who wouldn't survive in the world, I was certain I would terminate. But in the case of a nonfatal condition, in the case of Down syndrome, I hadn't reached a firm conclusion.

Or rather, the conclusion that I'd come to no longer felt firm. My mother was forty when she was pregnant with my brother, and she had an amniocentesis. "Would you have had an abortion if anything was wrong?" I'd asked her as a teenager. "Without a doubt," she told me. She said it with the same determination the words conveyed; for her the choice was clear. I had heard her certainty and internalized it; I had made it my own.

But now I was flooded with misgivings. We had tried for two years to get pregnant. Would I really end a pregnancy just because the child I was carrying was different from the one I'd pictured?

"I don't know," I said. "I just know that I'd want to know."

"I can transfer you to our front desk to schedule the amnio," Samantha offered. "They're scheduling ten days out."

I told her she could do that, and then, before she told me goodbye, she said, "I hope I haven't totally ruined your day!"

"No," I said, a fire in me burning her to hell. "It's okay."

I didn't move from my spot on the floor or replace the phone on its cradle. I just held it in my hand and looked at it for a moment before calling Kellie. My dog continued to nudge me. That thread of panic jolted me again as I waited for her to answer.

"What's up?" she asked.

I told her.

"Oh," she said. "Shit."

I could feel the silence fill the hundreds of miles between us.

"Do you want me to come home?" she asked.

I weighed my options.

Weeks earlier, when I had been nauseous and exhausted, I was often tempted to call in sick at work. But that seemed like a gamble. I could call in on Tuesday, but how did I know that Thursday wouldn't be even worse? I had made it to the end of my first trimester this way, never missing a day of work because I didn't want to use up all the grace I'd been allotted.

I felt the same way now. "Stay," I told Kellie. I would be visiting her this weekend anyways. "If we have to make a decision—if it comes to that—that's when I'll need you."

"I'm calling my mom," Kellie said. "She'll take you."

It hadn't occurred to me that I didn't need to go alone. I had automatically imagined driving myself to Seattle, walking myself through a day of appointments, and then driving myself home. Alone was my default mode. I thought about Geri with her platinum hair and square-framed glasses. I had been to her house dozens of times, but she still felt foreign to me, distant. I could refer to Geri as my mother-in-law, but it didn't feel completely true. Kellie and I weren't legally married; we still didn't have that option. The ambiguity of our relational status bled into our relationship. I wasn't sure who I was to her—if we were family to each other or not. It was possible that Geri and I had never had our own conversation aside from brief exchanges on the phone. Sometimes she'd call for Kellie and I would answer. Geri never announced herself, never opened with "Hello." Instead, she just launched into a line of questioning. "So, how'd it go?" she might ask me, her voice unmistakable.

"How did what go?" I'd ask, embarrassed to not know what she was talking about. "Oh," she'd say, realizing she had me and not her daughter. "You two are starting to sound alike."

The idea of Geri driving me in her car to Seattle was curious to me. I agreed to it because suddenly company didn't seem like such a bad idea. I agreed because I wanted Kellie to take care of me, even if she did so indirectly. I agreed because I liked the idea of our family relationships shifting, deepening even though I couldn't quite picture what they would become. I didn't quite feel safe, but I wanted to.

Because Geri hated driving and hated the freeway even more, she and her husband, Richard, picked me up early on a Wednesday morning. Nestled into the back seat, a passenger, I felt like I had so often as a child, in a state of surrender. I put on my seatbelt and rested one hand on the slope of my belly. Geri handed me a magazine she brought from home, a *Vanity Fair*. I flipped through and took comfort in a world so far from my own, in the smooth women wrapped in silk and gold, in the perfume samples that both transported and disgusted me. In the front seat, Geri flipped through her own magazine and commented to Richard on who was driving like an asshole and who had the nicest car. I took off my shoes and rested my feet on the console. I felt like a twelve-year-old, being taken by relatives to some tourist destination.

In the waiting room, the three of us sat side by side, Richard filling the chair on the end, Geri settled next to him, and I sat closest to the reception desk, all three of us divided by wooden armrests. I had a full day of appointments—an ultrasound, a consultation, and finally the amnio itself, with long waits in between, but we never discussed who would go where; we shared an understanding. Richard would wait all day in his seat, would rise occasionally to use the restroom or stretch his legs, while Geri would accompany me from room to room.

In the first room, Geri stood five feet away from me, and together we watched my baby move across the screen, watched it kick and punch and turn, both of us amazed and silent. Geri was there when the technician wiped the lube off my belly and handed me pictures, which I glanced at only briefly before stuffing them into my purse.

Geri followed as I was ushered into Samantha's office. She sat with me at the same round table where, months before, Samantha had said "I'm sorry" about a thousand times. Geri noticed how Samantha's face turned pink when I introduced her as my partner's mother, and Geri watched and listened as Samantha explained the process of amniocentesis, Samantha's eyes wandering around the room as she spoke, tracing the floor and the wall but never meeting my gaze. Geri commented as we returned to the lobby to wait some more, "That woman sure is *nervous.*"

"I have that effect on her," I said. Geri sighed and rolled her eyes.

Geri was still with me countless slow minutes later when a technician ushered me into yet another room and handed me a hospital gown. Geri averted her eyes as I undressed and put it on. As I sat on the edge of exam table covered in sterile paper, the utter silence of the room brought me to tears, and all of a sudden I was sobbing, choking on air. Geri didn't look away, but instead her own eyes filled with tears, and she reached for the tissue box by the sink and grabbed one for each of us. Geri became, in that moment, a member of my true family—not the family you map on a page that tracks bloodlines and legal marriage, but the short list you carry in your heart.

Later on the phone, Geri told Kellie (who reported back to me), "I just couldn't bear it, the sight of that needle—it must have been eight inches long."

But by the time the needle came, I had settled, eased into composure by a calm and confident doctor, an Asian American woman with cropped silver hair who spoke in measured tones, who treated the situation as normal and safe because, of course, this was something she did every day. I looked away as the needle entered my belly and thought about how it was strange that what I felt was a dull ache and not the sting of a puncture. When I looked again, the reservoir had filled with a yellowish fluid. As I left and the doctor explained that I would hear preliminary results within forty-eight hours, her assistant looked alarmed. "Oh, is she at risk for something?" the assistant asked, as if I weren't in the room, and the doctor nodded silently.

Before we left that day, I walked alone to the front desk to make a request. I leaned in and spoke to the receptionist in hushed tones. "This may be weird, but I have something to ask you," I said.

The receptionist cocked her head, ready.

"When my results come in, can you have someone else call me? Like, a different genetic counselor?" What I meant was *not Samantha*. "I just—if it's difficult news, I'd rather hear it from someone else."

The receptionist looked at me steadily. "I will make sure that happens," she said.

On the way home from the appointment, Richard pulled off the freeway so all of us could eat together. "Is this place okay?" he asked as he pulled into the parking lot of a steak house. I trailed him and Geri into the restaurant. We stood on tiled floors under bright lights as we waited for a table to clear. I had the same feeling I'd had on the car ride earlier, like I was not quite an adult. I leaned into that feeling. I was hungry. I never would have chosen a steak house for myself. That someone had chosen it for me, that I was about to sit with a big glass of ice water and order from a big laminated menu, brought me inexplicable comfort. When I was a child, going to a restaurant with my parents was a treat I anticipated for days. With Geri and Richard now, I ordered the kind of root beer that comes in its own brown bottle and a steak, well-done, that came with mashed potatoes and broccoli. Though I was mostly over my nausea, green vegetables still turned my stomach. Geri and Richard had ordered identical meals, and we sat together quietly, cutting up our steaks, taking comfort in mashed potatoes.

I got into bed that night the same way I had for most of the nights since Samantha's phone call: with a sense of dread that began in my stomach and radiated in all directions. I tried to sort out what I knew.

I knew that I believed in my right to make choices for my body. I knew also that having a child with Down syndrome would require a different kind of commitment than a typical child, that children with Down syndrome were more susceptible to a range of health problems, that they often required extra support like physical and speech therapy, and that few grew up to live independently.

But I knew that my fear had less to do with the extra time and financial investment a child with Down syndrome would require and more to do with social stigma. I'd grown up hearing and using the R slur as an insult, just as I'd grown up hearing and using "gay" as an insult. When I imagined introducing my new child to friends and family, and when I imagined this child having Down syndrome, I imagined a tension—a distance. I imagined people hiding their surprise and putting on fake smiles. I imagined them holding me at arm's length.

I tossed and turned, not quite wanting to face that truth

about myself. As a queer person, I knew the pain of being seen as an abomination. I knew the half smiles, the awkwardness. I knew the pain of being only half-accepted. As much as I wanted to avoid this pain, I didn't want to let it rule me.

There were other things I worried about. I could wrestle with my own misgivings, but I would also have to reckon with Kellie's. My stomach tensed with yet more worry as I thought about Rebecca and Daniel. We had never talked about what it would mean to make this kind of choice. The voices in my head chattered away until they reached a fever pitch.

And then, finally, as I lay tangled in my covers, I imagined a presence, distant from all the fearful voices—a blanket of light that hovered ten feet above me. I thought of my grandmothers, whom I knew, and the great-grandmothers whom I had never met, grandmothers who may never have approved of my life as it was but who had forged a path all the same. I thought of all of them before me, bearing children. I thought of their fears and imagined them alone in those fears, their husbands off at the bar, or off at sea, or sleeping beside them, likely unaware that women had worries of substance. Something about the thought of them, their worries and their lives, the fact that they had carried on and made it to the end and then departed, entering the realm of air and light—something about this was a comfort to me, bigger than the shape of my own fears.

I was washing dishes the following afternoon when the phone rang. My heart leapt at the noise. I braced myself before answering. I told myself it was too early for news.

The voice on the other end of the line was friendly and unfamiliar. "Hi, it's Megan from Prenatal Diagnosis," she said.

I pulled off my kitchen gloves and tossed them in the sink. I leaned against my counter. "Hi," I said.

"I'm calling with the preliminary results of your amniocentesis."

"Okay."

"All of your baby's chromosomes look fine. We see no sign of Down syndrome or any genetic abnormalities." Meghan paused and continued. "I have a note here that says you want to learn the sex of your baby?"

"Yes," I said. My heart pounded away. "Yes, I'd love to know that." I held my breath. It felt like a long moment as I waited for her to speak. I knew that Kellie had hoped so strongly for a girl. If given a choice, I would have chosen that too. That tiny hope was now like fly buzzing just beyond my peripheral vision: present but totally squashable.

"It says here that you're having a boy," she said.

I thanked her before hanging up the phone. I wished her a good day, my voice bright as if I could somehow convey the depth of my gratitude—because she'd relieved a fear, because she was not Samantha, because it was sunny outside and turning to spring.

I called Kellie, and then I called Geri. "A boy," I told each of them. "We're having a boy."

"Wait," Kellie said, breathless because she had run in from outside. "How do you know that already?"

"Well, shit," Geri said, exasperated from worry. "Thank god for that."

I made myself dinner and then spread out on the couch, one hand on my belly as I watched a movie. When I went to bed that night, I pulled the ultrasound pictures out from the drawer in my bedside table, and for the first time, I allowed myself to study them. The image was grainy, but the parts were clear: I could make out the edge of an ear and the slope of a backbone. The baby's hand, poised above his nose, formed a fist. I could make out every little finger.

A few days later, as I lay alone in bed on a Saturday morning, my phone rang. It was Rebecca and Daniel, sharing the line. I reached over and pulled up the window shade to let the light in while we talked.

"We heard you had a rough week," Rebecca said. Her voice was clear, like she was sitting next to me.

"Ugh," I answered. "I'm so glad it's over." I waited a moment before I confessed to them: "I was so worried too about what I'd tell you. Everything felt uncertain, and I didn't want to drag you into it."

"It would have been your decision," Daniel said. His voice, scratchy from sleep, conveyed no hesitation.

Rebecca jumped in to echo him. "It's your body and your family."

I sunk back into my pillows, feeling relieved all over again.

20
HOMECOMING / DISTANCE

Kellie was tan from months of working outside in the weather when she returned from the island. She was lean from having fed herself, from living on salad, banana chips, and tortillas with sriracha. When she came out of the shower, one towel wrapped around her hair, another around her waist, she suddenly looked tiny to me. "When did you get so little?" I asked.

"I'm still bigger than you," she retorted, but it wasn't true. I was still several inches shorter than her, but now I had at least twenty pounds on her. I was round and exploding. It wasn't just my belly or my breasts. Even my face was rounder; my arms were pillowy. When we held each other now, our fit was awkward, my belly an obstacle to be navigated, an active space between us.

In the months that Kellie had been gone, I'd held on to a fantasy that when she returned, she would be magically cured of her worries. All of her misgivings about becoming a parent would have disappeared, and we'd be like characters in a romantic montage—soft focus. She would rub my feet on the couch, tuck me in for naps, and whisper in my ear about all the things she couldn't wait for.

But Kellie didn't magically transform. Kellie remained Kellie. Her return meant I no longer had to haul bags of dog food from the car to the garage or vacuum my own car. Kellie took over the physical labor that went into caring for our house, and she placed a wide chair with a cushioned seat and wooden armrests at the kitchen table so that I would have a comfortable place to sit. But when it came to the baby, I sensed that any joy she may have felt was bound tightly in worry. I hoped I was wrong, and so I sometimes prodded her.

"How are you feeling?" I would ask.

"About the baby?"

I nodded.

"Scared," she answered.

I had hoped that the baby taking shape inside of me, the undeniableness of him, would dissolve Kellie's reluctance. But to Kellie the reality of this thing that got bigger week by week, this thing that would emerge in just a few months, squirming and crying—this thing was not reassuring. Sometimes, as he kicked and wiggled from inside of me, I took Kellie's hand and guided it to that spot. She waited for the next kick. So did I. Sometimes he responded with a gentle tap, discernible only to me. Sometimes he kicked on the opposite side, away from her hand. Sometimes he stopped kicking altogether.

"He doesn't like me," Kellie suggested.

I dismissed her, but her worry became my own. People always talked about fetuses like they were prescient, like their behavior in the womb revealed something about the person they'd become. I couldn't stop myself from thinking that way. For the whole of the second trimester, I craved potatoes so badly that I'd taken to making a plate of hash browns every morning. As I ate them, I wondered if my son would love potatoes, if he was dictating my cravings from the womb. And, likewise, I couldn't help but wonder if the baby was already telling us something about his relationship with Kellie, his second mother, if he was making it clear from the get-go that they wouldn't be an instant match.

I thought about fathers and biology; I thought about how if we were straight, if Kellie were a biological father, then perhaps I wouldn't worry about their connection—this child would be undeniably hers (his). There would be little to prove.

What were fathers allowed in this world, if not distance? I thought of my own father, who'd already had three children from a previous marriage when he met my mother. He was forty-four then—the same age Kellie was now. The dilemma of my mother's pregnancy was likely one he hadn't prepared for. Babies were far from his mind. He had lived for years in a one-bedroom apartment and seen his own kids once a month. His oldest child, at seventeen, was sent to live with my father for his final year of high school. This was his punishment for being a less-than-perfect teenage boy, to be banished from his small hometown and all the friends he'd known since childhood, to live instead with his father in an unfamiliar place. My father treated him like a roommate. They bickered over groceries and let the laundry overflow past the hamper.

This son, my half brother, had already graduated and moved out when my mother delivered the news of her pregnancy. A late period, a test, a tiny thing growing.

My father, I imagine, might have been relieved if my mother had decided to abort me. Perhaps he was relieved, for different reasons, that she decided to keep me. I imagine that for my father, my brother and I were a kind of security tax, a toll he paid to know that he had successfully resettled, secured a future that wasn't alone, that he had shed the bachelor's apartment for a more permanent home.

I don't say this to suggest he didn't love us or that he wasn't ultimately happy to have us. But we required an upfront investment of time and emotional energy and money. We filled the house with noise. We demanded things. There was no escaping us—not until our bedroom lights were extinguished could my father reclaim our house as his own. In general, I think my father cherished the idea of us more than flesh-and-bones reality of us—the crying babies who clung to his wife, the preteen with expensive orthodontia who sang loudly to the radio in her room, the teenager who hogged the family phone line. We orbited him, my brother and me.

But isn't that the way of things with so many fathers? We

exist on the peripheries of their lives. We are of them in the sense that we are built from their matter—a single sperm cell that meets an egg and then divides and grows. But that first cell is their only bodily contribution. We are not housed by them, borne by them. We do not depend on their blood to nourish us. My mother, pregnant with me, ate for two. She cut vegetables and imagined their vitamins crossing her placenta (an organ her body had made just for me) and entering my bloodstream. My father drank his morning coffee, cut his fried egg with a fork, and looked out the window. He didn't need to change. His body was, and would always be, his own.

I wondered to what extent the story of most fathers would also be Kellie's story. Kellie, who wouldn't grow this baby or nurse him. Kellie, who would always know that the baby carried my genetic code and not hers.

How deep would this knowing go? How important would it be?

Once, years ago, a friend of ours had noticed we both had blue eyes. "So cool," she said. "That means if you ever have kids, they will have blue eyes too." Kellie had laughed. I laughed too. "You're kidding, right?" I said. She looked at us blankly for a moment before realizing her error. "Oh," she said, joining our laughter. "I forgot." I loved her for forgetting. I carried that moment with me, always hoping that such forgetting was possible.

My hope was that Kellie herself, deep in her body, would

claim our baby, hold him against her, breathe away doubt. I hoped that this baby would come to know, as I did, the smell of her neck, the warmth of her skin. I hoped that she would know in return the smell of his head, that she would feel it in her body when he cried. I hoped they would be bound to each other, bodily, if not by DNA, then by the chemicals of love.

21
SETTING THE TABLE

When Geri offered to throw me a baby shower at her waterside home, I hesitated. I wanted to celebrate, but showers were the kind of ritual from the heterosexual world that felt utterly foreign to me. I thought about women in pastel dresses competing at blindfolded diaper changes or measuring the guest of honor's waistline. I thought about codes that enforced the gender binary, like blue and pink themes, conversations that leaned into stereotypes about boys versus girls, and the exclusion of men from the celebration.

It wasn't clear to me how easily these customs could bend to meet me and Kellie, two people who tensed every time someone generalized about how women liked to shop or how men were naturally more athletic.

I remembered that when Kellie and I had planned our wedding, along with the vulnerability of planning a ceremony that many outsiders would condemn, there was a sense of freedom. In rejecting the fundamental tradition of heterosexuality, every other tradition was ours to keep or do away with. Did we want to exchange rings? Yes. Did we need an ordained minister? No. Would we provide food and drink? Of course. Did we want to host a big rehearsal dinner? Nah, let's not.

In this way, being queer often meant making it up from scratch. But I wasn't sure what a queer baby shower would look like.

"It can just be a party," Geri assured me.

"Okay then," I said. A party we could do. We timed the shower to coincide with my own mother's summertime visit and saw it as a way to bring our community together—the grandmothers who lived on different coasts, the friends who had seen us through this endeavor so far and would help us through the next big transition.

My mother sat now in the back seat of my car as Kellie drove the endless straight road to Geri's. My mother would fly home in two days, and she wanted to know when she could return and meet the baby.

"Why don't you come once he's a month old?" I said.

My mother and I had already had this discussion, but it was clear she hoped my answer would change. "When I was pregnant with you," she warned me, "I was sure that I wouldn't need my mother's help. I told her not to come. And then I brought you home. You cried and cried and wouldn't stop crying. I had no idea what I had gotten into. The morning after your first night home, I called her and begged her to make the trip."

"I know," I said. I had heard this story before. "But we've got friends who can help and our house is just so small." I looked straight ahead at the tall pines on both sides of the road, but my mind's eye could picture my mother's face, fallen. I understood what she wanted: to hold this baby in her arms within moments of his arrival, to feel the weight of him, to cradle his head in the palm of her hand. This would be her first grandchild, and she wanted to claim him. She had waited for this moment.

But I couldn't give her that.

As a child, I had tried to be the companion my mother needed. She carried with her a grief and loneliness that often needed soothing. I had watched her struggle to keep herself together. She took pills to help her manage her feelings, which were big. The pills made her fuzzy—aloof but tender. They allowed her to carry on in a world that was often cruel and scary.

Her own childhood, I knew, had been painful. Her father drank in bars after work and came home in time to berate her younger brother before he passed out on the couch. My mother was left to pick up the pieces while my grandmother tried to keep the family afloat. She became the backup mother, the one who tended the house and made dinner while her own mother managed more distant threats: an absent husband, an empty bank account, a third child—unplanned for—on the way. It seemed to me that at some point, in the midst of all of this, my mom had found some kind of portal, a way of being half there and half gone, and this gone-ness would protect her. It seemed that she was fragile by nature, and rather than let her childhood harden her or toughen her, she escaped.

And so I tried to comfort her—when she broke into tears out of the blue, when she lamented her challenges at work or with my father. Like my mother had done for my grandmother, I tried to smooth the edges of her world by doing housework and caring for my brother.

As I entered adulthood, our relationship confused me. I wasn't sure where she ended and where I began. "You'll probably struggle with depression, just like me," she had said on several occasions, and I couldn't shake the feeling that she was handing down a sentence, that some part of her wanted me to know the pain she'd known, to be her companion in suffering.

Over the last few years, I'd made a practice of exploring the boundaries between us. "I don't think I want to talk about that," I said once when she began to confide in me about her marriage to my father. My mother looked taken aback, like I'd betrayed a promise.

I'd expected that once I'd laid boundaries and stood by them that I would feel a clear sense of relief and that my mother and I would find ourselves restored and companionable. But instead the air between us felt thicker and thicker. The more boundaries I set, the more distance I found I needed. And yet, the more distance I needed, the more I felt like a villain. My mother was a kind person who had loved me well. Holding her at arm's length often felt like an act of cruelty. I wasn't sure why I felt the need to, and yet I couldn't find another way.

This summer, our relationship grew even more complicated. For decades my mother had taken the same medications to manage her depression and anxiety. But recently, a doctor had prescribed a new set of drugs. The results so far had been alarming. In the weeks leading up to her trip, she had been sending me long, unpunctuated, stream-of-consciousness emails. This wasn't normal for her; my mother's career had been, in part, as a copy editor. Once, when I was in the fourth grade, I misspelled a common word in my homework. Let's say I left out the *e* in the word *homesick*. *Homsick*. My mother expressed concern that I couldn't spell something so simple. "I know how to spell it," I tried to convince her. "I just accidentally skipped the letter when I was writing. Doesn't that ever happen to you?"

She considered the question. "No," she said.

That exchange had baffled me so much that I had never forgotten it. Every time I missed a letter while writing by hand, I remembered.

That was partly why the unpunctuated emails worried me. But also, they were intimate in a way that made my heart race and my armpits sweat. Reading them was like being inside her swirling brain. In one of them, she imagined what my nipples would feel like after two weeks of breastfeeding: bleeding, cracked, and sore. I cringed. She had cc'ed my father.

In person, she was strangely frenetic—strangely, because

it seemed that she was trying to channel her wild energy into calming herself. On the first day of our visit, we had tried to have a conversation across my kitchen table. I served us cups of herbal tea. My mother declared that she was anxious, and I asked her what was on her mind. As she tried to explain it to me, she got flustered. "Stop!" she told herself, and then placed two hands around the mug I had given her. "Focus," she said, looking intently into the hollow of the cup.

"Are you—?"

"Don't interrupt," my mother scolded me. "I need to re-center." She inhaled through her nose. "Let me finish." I waited in silence for a full minute before she started talking again. When she spoke, I nodded along, hoping that if I pretended everything was normal, she might remain calm. But I wasn't calm; I was as flustered as she was. I was, in general and especially with my mother, an emotional sponge. If she felt something, I felt it too.

Having my mom in the delivery room or in my home right after the birth would spin me out of balance. She'd be there in my periphery as I breathed and pushed my baby into the world, as I swaddled him for the first time, as I learned how to latch him to my breast. When this baby arrived, I wanted him at the center of my attention.

It pained me now to hurt my mother, to imagine her own pain. I couldn't predict where that pain would land. Would she go home and cry into my father's arms? Would she complain to her therapist about how ungracious I was? Ungracious was exactly how I saw myself now as I looked out the passenger's window and reached for my water bottle. My mother had given me life, had delivered me into the world, and now I was denying her.

A few moments later, my mother's voice cut into the silence. "Will your donor be at the shower?" she asked. She didn't yet know our donor's name or what he looked like. She only knew that he existed, that he was a real person that we knew and not a number on file at a sperm bank.

Kellie and I shared a look.

"I think so," I said.

In truth, we knew that Daniel would be there. He and Rebecca had been the first guests we'd invited, and Rebecca had called us right back to say that she'd be out of town, but that Daniel would be there for sure. I felt worried for him, the donor at the lesbian baby shower. "How do you know Kellie and Jenn?" people might ask him. How would he answer? Would he feel a little bit like Peter Parker, his identity vulnerable, his spider suit hidden beneath plain clothes? I wished that I could protect him somehow, that I could orchestrate every interaction at the baby shower, but of course this was impossible. We were all simply at each other's mercy.

When we arrived, Daniel was already there, along with a few of our friends. My mother immediately approached him and began a conversation.

A heat wave had broken over the weekend, and the clouds had rolled in. The August air was cool now, though sticky. Our guest list was an odd one, combining family, our closest friends, and Geri's neighborhood friends—a group of older women I'd never met. No one ever spoke it, but I understood that Geri's friends were here to honor this one bright spot in what had been a dark year for Geri.

Her mother had died in November. Her death wasn't a surprise. She had lived with dementia for years, and Geri had gone through all of the rituals that so many children of declining parents go through. She had been the one to decide when it was time to move her into assisted living; she had visited weekly and tended to all the grooming rituals that the staff didn't have time for. She had dyed her hair, pulled her chin hairs, painted her nails. Geri had time to prepare for her mother's loss, and yet it was clear that she suffered for it. Tears leaked from her eyes any time her mom came up in conversation.

And then, two months later, Geri's only sister had died— suddenly—of a stroke. It happened on Christmas Eve, just hours after they had shared a holiday meal.

These weren't her only losses. Every few months, it seemed that Geri had a new funeral to attend, a friend who'd passed after a long battle with cancer or a sudden heart attack.

And so Geri's friends—who were strangers to me—arrived bearing onesies and blankets and board books. They hugged me and left me smelling like perfume. They hugged Kellie too and whispered to her about the great joy she was bringing to her mother. No one had ever expected Kellie to become a parent, and so this baby was a surprise gift.

Our crew of friends arrived in pairs and threes until the porch was filled with women my age—some of them in summer dresses, some of them in work pants—and an occasional husband and child. Victoria was there with her husband, her four-year-old child, and her new baby. Jo was there. Dee was there. My brother was there. Geri's friends and our friends didn't mingle much, but we coexisted happily. We shared the deck and dipped carrot sticks into ranch dressing and watched as boats moved through the water. Summer was ending; a baby was coming.

While my mother continued to talk to Daniel, I assessed the situation. I couldn't hear what they were saying, but both were smiling and Daniel leaned comfortably against a pillar. Maybe they didn't require my intervention.

I joined Victoria and a group of friends who were passing around her baby and cooing. Stella was already four months old. She had a perfectly round head covered in soft blond down and bright blue eyes. When I held her, I was surprised at her heft. She studied me intently as I positioned her on my hip. We had met a handful of times now, but it still felt like we were strangers to each other—pleasant but cautious. I wondered how it would feel to hold my own baby. Would it take us some time to know each other? Would he be a stranger too?

"Come with me," Kellie whispered in my ear. I handed Stella to the nearest set of outstretched arms. My mother was now talking to Geri as she moved from table to table, topping off every bowl with new pretzels. Kellie pulled at my hand and led me toward Daniel, who was alone now at the farthest corner of the deck. "Daniel has news," she whispered.

Just a few weeks earlier, Rebecca had called to tell us they were moving to the other side of the state, where the sun shone more often. Daniel had found a better job there. I assumed that Daniel's news now related to this move, that some other piece of their new lives had fallen into place. Maybe they were buying a house, I thought, or maybe Rebecca too had landed a job she wanted.

When we reached Daniel, Kellie hovered off to my side, grinning. We all stood there for a moment, our eyes moving through the triangle, Kellie, Daniel, and me.

"So?" I asked.

Daniel scanned the crowd behind me and leaned in. He spoke softly: "Rebecca's pregnant."

I looked at Kellie. I looked at Daniel. We all laughed. My cheeks flushed. A motor boat sped through the bay. Geri, who had disappeared inside, emerged now with a tower of cupcakes, and the group—Geri's friends and our own friends—began to assemble near the gifts. Geri waved me over to the seat of honor where I would begin the ritual of opening gifts for a human I had yet to meet.

As we left that day, my mother hugged Geri goodbye and said something about being in touch. "We'll see what we can work out," I heard Geri say. I wondered what they were talking about, but I didn't want to ask. As I closed Geri's front gate behind us, white balloons, attached with blue ribbon, bobbed up and down.

We had barely left Geri's driveway before my mother hit us with the question she'd been dying to ask. "Is Daniel the donor?"

"Yes," I answered, happy to offer the information now that we were safely in the car.

"I love it," she said. I was surprised by how much I enjoyed receiving her approval, by how much I needed it, in spite of the tension I carried.

As I rode along in the car, I remembered Kellie's warning to Rebecca and Daniel when they had first come over for dinner. "Be careful," she had told them. "You'll get pregnant too." Now, in spite of my surprise, I felt a sense of things falling into their places. "I sincerely hope you're first," Rebecca had answered that day. I had felt the same way—panicked that we might spend more years trying and failing, that Rebecca and Daniel would achieve a surprise pregnancy before our intentional one came through—if it ever came through.

But it was August now, and I was due in September. In my mind, if all went well, then there was no better scenario than the one we were living: our child would have an extended family on the other side of the state. It was still up in the air what we would call these folks. Would we call them aunt and uncle? Bio-family? Would we label these relationships at all? Or would we continue our lives as friends, tethered by something invisible and strong?

That night, Kellie and I stayed up talking in the dark. We talked about what it would mean to have two babies, biological half siblings, distant twins. Who would they be to each other? Instantly I pictured two tall, grown men sitting together on a porch somewhere, sharing a beer. I was happy for them, whoever they were, our imaginary future sons.

I was happy for me, too, to have stumbled into this situation. Only a couple of years earlier, I had insisted that I wanted to keep things as simple as possible. I had taken comfort in the idea of anonymity. But these new complications elated me. I felt like a plant, waking up to light, growing tendrils.

"Did you notice," I asked Kellie before we went to sleep, "when my mom was saying goodbye to your mom? Is she planning something?"

"I meant to tell you," she said. "I overheard her talking about staying with my mom when the baby's born. She doesn't want to wait a month."

"Are you serious?" I asked, but I didn't need an answer. It all made sense now. My blood pressure rose. My worry roused the baby, who began to nudge the inside of my right hip.

———

Two weeks after our baby shower, I sought the counsel of a therapist I had once seen regularly. I sat on her velour couch, rested my feet on her ottoman, and told her I was there to get advice about my mother. She sat across from me in a desk chair—a yellow legal pad in her lap and a Portuguese water dog sleeping at her feet. I hadn't seen her in over a year, but nothing in her office had changed. "What's up?" she asked me.

I did my best to explain the events of the last few months—the emails, the negotiations over her visit, my fear that she would show up for my baby's arrival even though I had asked her to wait. Whenever I spoke of my mother, my breathing got shallow. "I feel crazy and mean when I'm around her," I said.

My therapist listened with her eyes focused on me, her lips slightly pursed—it was a listening face I remembered well. I expected her to give me a lecture about boundaries, for her to prescribe some sort of confrontation where I would lay down the law and live with the fallout. I dreaded this advice, because if she told me this, then I would have to do it, and I didn't want to. I didn't want to hurt my mother.

"It sounds like she knows she can't stay with you," my therapist said. "So if she comes in spite of your wishes, can your brother run interference?"

"Maybe?" I said. My cheeks were hot. I tried to imagine Nick running my mother on errands or taking her out to dinner. He could keep her busy for an hour or two, no doubt, but what if she stayed for weeks? I could feel the furrow in my brow grow deeper.

"Jenn," my therapist said calmly, and I looked up.

She met my gaze and held it steadily. "At the end of a day, it's a free country and your mom can get on a plane if she wants.

You can't control that. And here's the beautiful thing about having a baby: everyone gets a seat at the table."

She paused, and I sat there, playing that sentence over in my mind. *Everyone gets a seat at the table.* I pictured a literal table, a long wooden one with places set and a feast laid out in the middle. There were pies and meat and bowls of purple grapes. I pictured linen napkins and shining silverware. And I pictured my mother as one guest among many. It didn't matter if her new medications left her off-balance, if she talked in circles now and had trouble listening. It didn't matter that we had history between us that made our time together fraught. I mean, yes, these things mattered—they would always matter, but other things mattered more. It mattered more that I was bringing a new person into the world, and that person would have his own connection to my mother—one that was blessedly separate from the one that she and I had.

I could offer her that: a seat at the table.

———————————

A few days after I met with my therapist, my mother called. We had emailed but not spoken since her return home. Her emails, gradually, had become more measured and coherent. Her new doctor, she reported, had changed her medication. On the phone, her voice was calm and untroubled. "I'm starting to feel like myself again," she said.

"It seems like you are," I agreed.

We made small talk about the weather and about the last weeks of my pregnancy. And then I tried to broach the subject of her visit. "So, were you thinking about coming out and staying with Geri?" I asked.

My mom was ready for the question. "I'll come when you want me to," she said. "I know you have lots of help. I'm just excited."

"I know you are," I said. When I hung up the phone, I felt new room in my chest.

22
LEGALITIES

"Do me a favor and get a lawyer." Dr. Katz's request followed me during the last months of my pregnancy. Kellie and I had always planned to make her a legal parent, but the doctor's show of concern that day in her office had added some urgency. It was true that I trusted Daniel and Rebecca to honor our agreement. I couldn't imagine any circumstance where Daniel would suddenly decide he wanted to sue us for custody. I also trusted both Kellie's family and my own—there was no relative on either side who would, for instance, decide if I died that Kellie had no right to raise our child. Or at least I didn't think so.

But there were two other things I knew. Of all the people who wound up in some kind of epic legal battle over their children, very few of them ever saw it coming. And I knew that our status as a queer couple made Kellie's role extra vulnerable, tenuous at best in the eyes of the law.

There was no easy way to make Kellie a legal parent. If we

had been a straight, married couple who had conceived with donor sperm—even if that sperm had come from a community member—no one in the delivery room would have asked any questions. My husband's name would automatically be listed as father. But in our actual circumstance, Kellie's name would be nowhere on our child's birth certificate, even though we could both attest without hesitation that we were a couple and that we had conceived this child with the intention of raising it together. If we wanted Kellie to have any legal rights, we would have to buy them.

Even as of this writing, when all fifty states and the federal government recognize gay marriage, and when most states have provisions that allow a nonbiological parent to appear as the second parent on the birth certificate, LGBTQ+ advocacy groups uniformly recommend second-parent adoption as a necessary step to protect the intended family relationships. As Cathy Sakimura, family law director of the National Center for Lesbian Rights, told *The New York Times*, "You can be completely respected and protected as a family in one state and be a complete legal stranger to your children in another."[34]

And so, Kellie and I pursued a second-parent adoption.

There were lawyers who specialized in LGBTQ family law, but they all lived in Seattle and seemed like designer lawyers, ones that might cost us two or three times what we would pay if we were willing to trust someone local and unspecialized. We asked a friend of a friend, who had a law degree, if she might know anyone who could help us. She thought about it for a minute, shrugged, and said, "I don't know—my neighbor, maybe?"

Her neighbor, it turned out, practiced family law from a small A-frame building less than a mile from where we lived. She was a hefty woman who shook our hands with a firm grip and sat us down on a leather sofa. She eyed my belly.

"I had twins," she said. "They're in college now. You'll probably breastfeed, right?"

I nodded.

"You're in for it. I never left my armchair. I just sat there with one kid on each boob and a Diet Coke on each armrest." I could picture her filling an armchair, shirtless. Strangers offered up these sorts of details readily now, anytime I was with Kellie, never when I was alone. They struck me as the speaker's way of compensating for our difference, an effort to offer something vulnerable and weird since we—because we were visibly queer and expecting—had shared something vulnerable with them. Being gay sometimes felt similar to conversing with a person who had just walked in on you in the bathroom. You might pretend together that everything is normal, but it feels like they've got something on you.

Our lawyer spread a bunch of paperwork across her desk and walked us through the process. Daniel would need to sign away his paternity rights. That part was easy: one standard form and a notary stamp and he would no longer be the father. We could just drop it in the mail with some instructions. Making

Kellie the second parent would be harder. It would involve not just a pile of paperwork, but two visits from a social worker. A "home study," it was called. A stranger would come to our home to study us.

She wrote the name of a social worker on a sheet of paper. "I know the whole thing is stupid," she said. "But she's one of you, so she won't give you any trouble."

"One of us—does that mean she's gay?" I asked Kellie on the ride home.

"Fuck if I know," she said.

The social worker was apologetic too. "I'm sorry I have to do this," she said. She sat at our kitchen table, which we had cleared off in preparation for her visit. We had cleaned for her, like people do, even though it struck me as silly. Would it matter if there were a pile of bills on the kitchen table? Would some dog hair on the floor indicate that we were unfit to care for our own child?

With her permed blond hair and floral dress, the social worker didn't immediately set off my gaydar. She asked us how we felt about spanking, how heavily we drank, and if we'd ever been convicted of any felonies. And then, as she was packing up her briefcase, she suggested that we all get together once the baby was born. "My daughter's three," she said. "She doesn't know any other two-mom families."

My heart sank a little when she said it. Her voice was tinged with loneliness. She seemed like a person I would have been happy to meet in any other context. I wanted to know some other two-mom families too. But I didn't feel like being friends with the social worker I'd never asked for, the person who would soon be sending me a bill for visiting my home and writing a report that assessed whether or not I'd be an adequate parent. I didn't want to feel that way about it, to transfer my frustration with the system onto her, an agent within the system who wanted to help us. I didn't want to, but I did.

At the end of the day, we spent nearly as much on making Kellie a legal parent as we would have spent on a round of IVF or a down payment on a foreign adoption. I had planned on dropping a thousand or two on these legal arrangements; I had never planned to pay ten thousand. In my mind I enumerated all the reasons we were lucky: We both had jobs that paid enough and our home carried a mortgage lower than what most people paid for rent. Our community had come through with sperm before we had gone into deep debt. I had health insurance to cover the costs of my pregnancy. I knew for a fact that there were plenty of queers who became parents without any of these benefits. They sourced sperm on the fly and trusted love and community to protect them, not the law. Even ten thousand dollars later, I still wasn't sure that I trusted the law to protect me, but I'd rest a little easier knowing I'd done what I could.

23
DELIVERY

I was exactly one week past my due date when I flopped onto bed next to Kellie and moaned, "I'm so done." Earlier that day an acquaintance had told me, "You'll know when you're about to go into labor because all of a sudden you'll have lots of energy."

"Well, then it's not going to be today," I told her, "because I feel like shit." As I hoisted myself into bed now, the weight of my belly felt impossible; it was like trying to move through the world with an anvil tied to my waist. I was so tired I was angry. All of my sensory nerves were firing at once. I turned on my side, exhaled, and let myself fall into sleep.

Just after midnight, something woke me. An ache. It was an ache I recognized from nearly twenty years of menstruating, the ache of my uterus contracting, like a towel being wrung out. Outside in the dark, an owl hooted. My ache subsided. Stillness. The owl hooted again. Kellie slept. I wouldn't wake her, I decided. Not yet. Instead, I tuned into my baby's motion.

I let his kicks and swipes reassure me. He was still in there, alive, moving the same way he did yesterday and the days before that. I wondered what it felt like to be the thing inside of that contraction. Did it feel like a squeeze, a push? Could he sense that the life he'd known up until now—the life of darkness and saline, of muffled sounds, of practiced underwater breaths— was about to end? That he would be pushed into a world of light and air, transformed forever?

Another contraction, 12:22 a.m. I tracked time on Kellie's alarm clock, the digits glowing red. The pain was remarkably bearable. Within the pain, I could feel the promise of the pain subsiding. It felt reliable and even. Cool air came through the cracked window. One more at 12:32 a.m. The ache returned, a small but grinding force, and with it, a trickle down my leg. I stood up. More fluid—more than I could contain.

"You okay?" Kellie asked me, her voice muffled by her pillow. She asked me this every night when I got up to pee, her sleep brain poised for my labor. Every night I laughed and told her I was fine. "I think my water broke," I said this time.

"Are you sure?" she asked.

I walked to the bathroom, my gait wide so I could avoid the soaked-through crotch of my boxer shorts. I turned on the light. On the floor I could see a trail of water. I sat on the toilet to pee. In the toilet bowl, I left behind an array of excretions: urine and a fresh streak of blood—but also tiny bits of old blood that looked like ground chalk. I had never read about this, about the blood and the matter one's body released in early labor. I worried, but the baby was now poking me with all his limbs at once. I could feel heels and elbows and knees. He was undeniably alive.

Kellie appeared in the doorway. She assessed the water on the floor. "Your water really did break."

"You didn't believe me?"

"I didn't know." She grabbed a handful of rags from the shelf and began to clean.

On my way back to the bedroom, I turned the kitchen light on. There, on the linoleum floor, in a small puddle of water, lay what must have been my mucous plug. As I stood there inspecting it, grossed out and amazed, Kellie joined me. "Wow," she said. She examined her rag.

"Don't," I said. "I'll get it." I grabbed a handful of toilet paper and winced as I scooped it up. Another contraction came, and I grimaced.

"How will we know when it's time to go?" Kellie asked me.

I washed my hands and called the midwife, who told me to go back to bed. She didn't need to see me until my contractions came at five-minute intervals. "Rest while you can," she told me. It was just after one in the morning.

I slept between contractions—the rhythm of it was easy. I spooned next to Kellie and dozed. When the tension in my body woke me, I squeezed her hand. She announced the time. 1:10 a.m., 1:20 a.m., 1:30 a.m. My body was strangely precise.

The owl hooted on. Cool air came through the crack in the window. Outside, there was nothing but darkness. We were moving through that darkness, sleeping and waking, contracting and relaxing, like swimming laps in a pool.

When the clock read 6:00, when there was a small edge of light in the sky, Kellie rose from the bed. "I'm making coffee," she announced. Without her, the room felt charged and empty. I heard the whir of the coffee grinder. My uterus folded—out of nowhere, a new kind of contraction, deeper and longer. I gripped the bed rail. I moaned. It was 6:07 a.m.

In the car, on the way to the hospital, my baby continued to nudge me from the inside. I tried to allow myself to feel joy. I told myself I would meet my baby today. But I doubted. It seemed so abstract, so unreal. This thing that had been squirming and kicking inside of me, would it really see light? Would it really come out of me alive and whole?

In the prenatal yoga class I had attended, the instructor asked us to introduce ourselves and check in at the beginning of each class. Every time a woman announced that she was planning a home birth, she got a round of cheers from the instructor and the other students. In private, the instructor recounted to me what she hated about hospital births. She had never birthed in a hospital, nor attended a hospital birth, so she couldn't tell me anything specific about our local hospital where I planned to deliver, but she was convinced they were all the same. They would pressure me into a C-section if my progress was slow, she warned me. They would insist I get an epidural even if I didn't want one.

I had my own concerns about the hospital. Every woman in my yoga class had been straight and married. At our birthing class, Kellie and I were conspicuously the only queer couple. In fact, I had walked into the first session alone while Kellie parked the car, and the instructor asked if I had a birthing partner joining me. "She's parking the car," I said, happy for the chance to prepare the room for our difference. "Oh," the instructor had said. "Is it your mother?"

I was worried about how the hospital would receive us. I didn't want to be pushed into a C-section or an epidural, that was true. But I worried also about how things would go if the attending nurse, for instance, wasn't fond of us or if any of the staff, consciously or not, treated Kellie as if she didn't quite belong there.

But it had taken me years to conceive this child, and there was never a moment of my pregnancy where I took the desired outcome—a live, healthy baby—for granted. I chose a hospital birth to keep my bases covered, had selected a midwife rather than an obstetrician in hopes that I could keep invasive interventions to a minimum, and I prayed that the social dynamics wouldn't be a shitshow.

The maternity ward was in the basement of the hospital. Bright fluorescent lights bounced off linoleum floors. The hospital had speakers wired to broadcast the melody of "Twinkle Twinkle Little Star" each time a child was born. The tune was playing as Kellie guided me inside, one hand on my back. "It's a busy morning here," the receptionist told us as she walked us to our room. "Barometric pressure rose. Lots of babies coming." I pictured newborns falling from the sky like rain.

Just inside our room, a nurse named Dotty greeted us. She was sinewy and tall, with cropped platinum hair and pink lipstick. She was the same age as our mothers.

"This is my partner," I said. I didn't want to let anyone ruin this day by asking Kellie if she was my mother.

"Does your partner have a name?" Dotty asked.

Kellie used both of her hands to shake Dotty's.

I crossed the room so I could brace myself against the side of the hospital bed. A big one was coming. I let the pain pass through me. I bit my lips so I wouldn't cry out. "You can make noise," Dotty told me. "Scream. You won't scare us."

"What radio station do you want?" Dotty asked once I stood up again.

"I don't know," I said. "Whatever you want." Dave Matthews was playing in the background.

"Honey," she said, "you're working harder than any of us. You choose."

"Is this the Mountain?"

Dotty nodded. The Mountain was our local station that recycled all the cheesy rock songs from the '90s.

"Keep it on." I knew that some couples made special playlists for their day, but I was content to just hear music I didn't mind—Pearl Jam, Alanis Morisette—music I'd been hearing in the background for all of my adult life. When I was twenty years old, before I knew Kellie, I used to bake wedding cake layers all day in a warehouse. The Mountain blared from a boom box that was covered in flour and splattered frosting. To hear it now, a dozen years later, as I attempted to enter motherhood, was comforting.

Dotty gave us a tour of the room. Next to the bed sat a bright green gymnastic ball. "Try leaning on that when the next one comes. Some people like it." The next one came. I dropped to my knees, spread my arms over the ball and let myself moan. "That's right," Dotty said. Kellie knelt beside me, her face trained on mine. She was in the moment, witnessing, serious about her job. It was the kind of undivided attention I craved every day of my life.

"Let me know when you're ready for the tub," Dotty said, directing us to the bathroom. I saw my own face in the mirror. I was flushed, and my hair was frizzy from the moisture of my sweat. "It's best to get in when you get to that point where the pain is unbearable."

"I'm not there yet," I said.

Dotty leaned over to turn on the faucet. "Let's just have it ready."

"Shit," I said, as the next one took hold. This one was worse than the one before. Riding it out was like diving into a wave and letting it carry me to shore. I emerged from the pain breathless but whole. "I'm ready for the tub," I said.

Every so often, Dotty knelt beside the bath with her Doppler machine. She held the probe against my belly, and our baby's heartbeat came through the monitor as a series of staticky bumps. With each contraction, the heart rate markedly slowed. It paused for a moment and then sped as if to make up for those lost moments. I looked at Dotty. "He might have the cord around his neck," she said. "I know how scary that sounds, but it's common."

I looked to Kellie.

"It's okay," she told me. "We're in the right place."

The bathwater was tepid and pink from my blood. "I want out," I told Dotty.

Dotty helped me out with a white bath towel. That towel was my outfit now. It didn't cover much. As Dotty draped it over my shoulders she told me, "Don't start pushing yet. When you start to feel like you've got to take the biggest crap of your life, you let me know and then we'll check you."

"I might already feel that way," I said. It was hard to tell. I felt pressure everywhere. I tried not to look down. My belly looked strange, no longer the round high bump I had watched grow over the last months. Now it seemed low, lopsided; it was actively transforming. That there was a large, live thing working its way out of me was a reality I didn't want to face directly. If I thought about it, I would think of all the things that could go wrong. How does anyone survive the birth canal? I wondered.

I lay naked on the hospital bed so that Dotty could check my cervix.

"You're at ten centimeters," Dotty said. "You can push."

She set up a birthing stool, a white plastic seat shaped like a crescent moon. Dotty arranged the towel over my shoulders. Beneath it I was naked and sweating, my breasts hanging low. I wanted to hide them, but my clothes were in a pile on the floor, and they seemed to belong to a different world. I was an animal now. There was no going back.

When I leaned forward, I could rest my hands on the bed rail. With the next contraction, as I pushed, I gripped that rail and used it for leverage. Kellie stood to my left, breathing with me, one hand on my back.

The contractions came steadily, and with each one I pushed. I wasn't sure if I was doing it right. All I could tell was that the pain was moving through me, and now instead of breathing through it, I was pushing into that pain. My body was one big column of pressure. When each contraction eased, the pressure below remained. There was a baby in my birth canal, stretching me in all directions. There was no relief from that.

Dotty had hooked me up to a monitor, so the baby's heartbeat was broadcasting through the room. It competed now with my moans, and with the radio, which was now playing "Crazy on You." The baby's heart rate kept slowing and then recovering with each contraction.

"Don't worry," Dotty told me.

I worried.

"We made it this far," Kellie reminded me.

I took comfort in the idea of a C-section, of being wheeled away to some other room and being cut open, my baby rescued from me.

I looked at the clock. It was almost noon. I had been here for nearly four hours. This surprised me. Time had been strange all morning, not marked by minutes but by the rhythm of pain and relief.

I pushed again. "Your baby has hair," Dotty said. She motioned to Kellie to come look. Kellie crouched next to Dotty so she could see, but the baby had already slipped back inside of me. He wasn't crowning yet, just surfacing and hiding. The next contraction pushed the very top of his head back into view. When Kellie saw what Dotty had seen, she laughed. "Look at that," she said.

"He really has hair?" I asked.

"A ton of it," Kellie answered. "Dark, like yours."

I had always pictured a baby with a smooth, downy head, never one with hair. Already he was his own.

The midwife entered, which meant they were getting ready to catch the baby. Dotty must have had some way of signaling that we were ready, but it felt like telepathy. She and Dotty laid out a sheet on the floor beneath the birthing stool and, on top of it, a small steel basin. It occurred to me that this signaled the end of my delivery. They were getting ready to catch my baby. I looked at the clock again. I'd been pushing for forty minutes. I'd been in the hospital for less than five hours. I was worried, though. Somehow, it didn't seem like enough. That I was minutes away from meeting my baby felt impossible to me. I wasn't sure I'd worked hard enough yet.

"You're almost there," Dotty told me. "But this last part is tricky. You have to push him around the pubic bone." She held a mirror beneath me so that I could see. With the next push, I could glimpse the top of his head, could see his thick, black hair for myself. His heart rate slowed again and then started. "Try three more pushes," Dotty said.

I tried three more pushes and then another three. There was no way I could have done a dozen more, but I could do three and three and three and three.

Hours passed this way. I kept waiting for someone to stop me, to comment on how futile this was, but no one did. At one point, the midwife instructed me to lie on the bed with my knees in the air. With each contraction, each push, Dotty held my hands and pulled me toward her. The position was dynamic. I was pushing, she was pulling. But after six contractions like this, the baby remained in the same position, and Dotty wiped sweat off her brow. "That's about all I can do," she huffed. I wanted to apologize. We had gone through six contractions that way, and it hadn't occurred to me a woman in her midsixties might find it strenuous to brace the weight of a grown and pregnant woman.

I returned to the birthing stool, discouraged. How long would they let me labor like this?

On the monitor, my baby's heart continued to mark the rhythm of our birthing, his heartbeat steady between contractions, silent as I pushed, fast as I released. I stayed tuned into that rhythm, grateful that such a thing could be measured. But in this last contraction, Dotty must have heard something on the Doppler—a long stall—that I hadn't noticed. "Baby's tired," she said to the midwife, who nodded in agreement.

"Baby's tired." To me it sounded like: *Baby's dying.*

The midwife approached me and crouched so we were at the same level. It was the first time since my arrival at the hospital that we'd met eye to eye. Her name was Julie, and for the course of my pregnancy, I had seen her for half of my appointments. She and a colleague ran a practice together, and I had hoped that her partner would be the one on call when I went into labor. The partner was six feet tall, dark-haired, and charismatic. Julie, on the other hand, had honey-colored hair that blended with her skin tone. She rarely raised her voice above a whisper. And in this moment, as she looked me in the eye and explained to me my options, I realized that charisma is not what you need from your midwife when you're trying to birth a child.

"So," Julie explained, "your contractions have slowed down. If you want to keep pushing, you can. We can try a dose of

Pitocin and keep monitoring your baby's heart rate. Or, you might consider if you want a vacuum assist."

"I want the vacuum," I told her. I knew that there were risks. I refused though to think about what they were; I pushed them to the back of my mind before they could come into focus. I was convinced this baby wouldn't leave my body without help. If this was what it would take, so be it.

Dotty returned me to the bed in preparation. With the next contraction, as we waited for the doctor to arrive, she and Kellie urged me to push. "You can do this!" they shouted and Kellie squeezed my hand. I knew what they were thinking—that this incentive, the doctor on the way, would help me push this child into the world. I didn't believe them. I pushed. That same one-inch of my baby's head revealed itself again and then retreated.

When Kellie and I remember that day, we swear that Dr. Bell showed up in shorts as if he had been called in from the golf course. It seems that this memory can't be accurate, that he must have arrived like any doctor, in khakis and scrubs, and yet we share it. He put on latex gloves, and, as he prepared the vacuum, the midwife coached me. "It's not time to relax yet," she explained. "When you have your next contraction, you need to give it your all. That's how we're going to get this baby out of you."

"Okay," I said, but I didn't trust myself to do it. Julie had already informed me that my contractions were slowing down. It was easy now to see my body as incapable, a failure.

Dr. Bell was ready. Dotty was ready. Julie was ready. My

next contraction came. I pushed into it with everything I had, even though what I had was less than nothing. I didn't care that it might not be enough—I pushed as if it was; I pushed knowing that the doctor was on the other side, helping me deliver. I pictured the baby's head splitting me open to be free. I was fine with that. They could stitch me up later. I was fine with whatever it took. Deliver him from me, please, I thought. Deliver him in one fell swoop.

The contraction ran long—it was one long line of action, me pushing, the doctor pulling, an extraction. I felt nothing precise. I could not tell you when the baby left me; I could only tell you that when my pushing ended, I felt, in addition to the bright red pain, a sense of relief. And also: action swirled around me. There was a creature just beyond me, new to the world. He was being tended to.

In every birthing video I had watched over the last three months, there was a horrifying moment—horrifying to me—where the baby came out blue and silent. There was a long pause before the first breath and the cry. I had watched these movies over and over and coached myself: be ready for that moment. Be ready for that short but eternal moment of waiting.

I told myself that now in the hospital room.

And then I heard my baby cry. Kellie held him as the midwife cut the cord. I strained to lift my head, but I could not yet glimpse him. Instead I saw four adult bodies, huddled over the brand new thing, consulting.

Finally Kellie brought him to me, wrapped in a blanket. "He's really cute," she whispered. I was crying. She laid him on my chest, his bare skin against mine. I was surprised by the weight of him, the warmth of him. He was already as much a person as he was a baby. He looked at me with bright eyes. I had imagined that my baby would come out squinting and snuffling, born but not quite present. But my child looked at me now as if I too were surprising.

"Hi," I whispered, over and over.

As I held him, Julie explained that they needed to stitch me up. She and Dr. Bell leaned over my pelvis. I felt the occasional pricks of a needle, but mostly I just watched my baby. Forty minutes passed before it occurred to me that it was strange that they were still stitching.

I've seen pictures of women after labor where they look vibrant, like they just returned home from a brisk walk. In the pictures of me after my birth, I look pale and exhausted, my hair sweaty and matted. I couldn't walk unassisted. Dotty brought me a brown plastic cup with orange juice over ice. I sipped it through a straw. Then she helped me to the bathroom and stood beside me. She wanted me to pee, even though it struck me as the last thing I wanted to do. My body felt exploded. It was all one mess of radiating pain. I sat on the toilet for minutes, trying to locate the right muscles. Dotty had witnessed me naked, pushing, and moaning, she had seen me from all angles, and now she stood by me at the toilet, patiently waiting to hear the trickle of my pee.

Of all the interactions I'd had with the medical, fertility, and birthing communities, this one—my son's delivery—was by far the most competent. In the hours I spent birthing my child and the two days that followed, my queerness was nearly invisible to me. To some extent, this might have been lucky. Dotty struck me as an exceptional human, and she may just have easily been assigned to another family that morning. It's possible that someone else might have made us feel unwelcome, and if that were the case, my memory of my son's delivery would have been a stinging, rueful one, my joy at his arrival tempered by the familiar feeling of being ushered to the margins. Though it didn't happen that way, I can picture it.

And it's possible that the urgency of delivery eliminated some of the room for missteps and awkwardness that were so common in other interactions. With all of us—mothers, midwife, doctor, nurse—focused on the same imminent goal, it felt natural to coalesce.

But it strikes me also that the hospital itself must have been competent in ways that were meaningful to us. Besides Dotty, there were many other nurses who touched our family over the two days we were there, and not one of them made a bad assumption or asked about the baby's father. And so, in those first moments—for once—I had the luxury of tending only to my baby and my own self-care. I was not distracted by the persistent bruise of being othered.

"Everybody wants to meet the baby," Kellie told me once I'd resettled in the bed. She held the baby with her left arm, her fingers spread wide to cradle his head. She looked like she'd been holding newborns all her life.

"Really?" I asked. This hadn't been our plan. I had imagined we'd keep the baby to ourselves until morning. Articles on transitioning into motherhood had advised me that this would be what I wanted, and I had believed them. I had read that I would be in some kind of animal state, tired and protective, baring my teeth at intruders. But when I checked in with myself, that wasn't how I felt. My body was spent, but my heart was expanding. I wanted to let the world in.

They all arrived together: Geri and Richard, Kellie's brother Ronnie and his two teenage sons. Someone had managed to pick my brother up along the way. Kellie's father came, and her Grandma Betty, her hair stiff and white, her pink lipstick fresh. The baby was asleep still, swaddled in a blanket, wearing his standard-issue newborn cap.

Geri approached us first, and as she glanced at his face and then at mine, she instantly burst into tears. So did I. We looked at each other, laughing and crying and wiping at tears, and I understood that for both of us that moment held the ghosts of other moments—the ghosts of Geri's countless losses over the past months, the ghosts of my two years of failures, the ghost of that giant needle poking through the layers of my belly just a few months before. And now here he was, undeniably present in spite of all of it: this perfect sleeping infant. He was so real, you could hold him. We passed him from mother to grandmother, from grandmother to grandfather, from grandfather to stepgrandfather to great-grandmother to uncle to uncle, while teenage cousins looked on, and then back to another mother—Kellie—where he stayed.

24
BECOMING FAMILY

*In the fourth century BC, Aristotle proposed a theory of repro-*duction that would persist for thousands of years. It's a theory that, while scientifically inaccurate, still informs some of our cultural thinking about parenthood.

According to Aristotle, the man, via intercourse, planted his seed in the woman's womb. The woman's menstrual blood nourished that seed and allowed it to grow. She provided the habitat, he the genetic content. The resulting child was of the father, nourished by the mother.[35]

In other words, when it came to parenthood, the woman's essential role was to nurture what the man had planted within her. Women, according to this theory, produced no gametes. Their eggs were still undiscovered.

To father was to simply provide the material—a temporary, momentary job. Fathering was ejaculating.

To mother was to care for. This job was ongoing,

never-ending. Her care began at the moment of conception and continued into adulthood and beyond. Mothering was nurturing.

Moreover, the child was seen as the genetic product of the father only. Consider a flower that grows from a seed. The soil is essential, but it is secondary, in service to the seed. Through Aristotle's lens, a genetic connection made a man a father, but had nothing to do with motherhood.

When Kellie and I came home from the hospital, our house felt strangely quiet and bare. In the days preceding delivery, Kellie had cleaned and organized as a way of getting ready for the baby, and our house was now unusually tidy. We sat on the couch with our sleeping baby and admired him. We smoothed his hair so that it crested at the center of his forehead, Napoleon style, and then we smoothed it to the side. We said his name— West—over and over, trying to teach ourselves the word for this new being. Every so often he twitched. I had the sense that our world was about to transform, that the quiet of the first newborn days was temporary.

In the days that followed, I roamed the house in mismatched pajamas and snacked on casseroles that friends had brought over. I nursed the baby and rocked the baby and watched the baby while he slept. Meanwhile, Kellie and Jesse—the contractor who had long ago declined to be our donor—built walls around our back porch to create a mudroom for our house. In the months leading up to our baby's birth, we'd agreed that our dogs would need such a room, a place set away from a baby who would one day be crawling and drooling and grabbing. All day now I heard Kellie and Jesse's hammering and muffled conversation.

In this way, we entered parenthood. I was the full-time nurser and the guardian of sleep; Kellie was the builder, the house-maintainer. At night, the baby slept between us.

———————

The idea that paternity is primarily a genetic contribution, that a father's role is simply to provide the seed, is a very stubborn one. An absent father is still considered a father. When we use the word *fathering*, we are usually referring to the physical act of conception, while the term *mothering* more often describes the act of tending-to. When a father takes on some of the active parenting tasks, when he drives the kids to school or makes them breakfast, we often refer to these acts as "helping," as if he were doing tasks assigned to someone else. "He's a good father," I've heard people say, bemoaning a wife's lack of gratitude. "He helps."

"Who's the dad?" is a question I get asked from time to time when people learn that my son has two mothers.

The idea that my son doesn't have a dad, that it is indeed *possible* to not have a father, is a hard thing for people to wrap their minds around. Even for me, it creates a kind of cognitive dissonance. When I say that my child has no father, I feel like I'm not telling the whole truth.

By the time Rebecca and Daniel met our baby, they had a baby of their own. We met them at a pizza place on a weekday afternoon. They had come to town to visit family—to stay with Rebecca's sister and brother-in-law—and meet up with longtime friends who wanted to see their new child. At the time, our relationships to each other still tentative and undefined, we counted more as friends than family.

I remember that meeting in fragments, like bits of color held up to the light: Trays of half-eaten pizza. Plastic cups filled with ice water. Rebecca holding her newborn against her, a burp cloth draped over her shoulder, her baby's feet naked, the creases in his chubby ankles. My own baby old enough to crane his head and look around with wide eyes and a two-tooth smile. All of us in constant motion—standing to rock the baby; sitting to feed the baby; slipping into the bathroom to change the baby's wet diaper. We passed our babies from one parent to the other and then across the table, trading babies, each of us taking a turn to feel the heft of each new addition, to look him in the eyes and greet him.

I remember it this way: we were neither distant nor close, neither awkward nor easy. We'd all been remade by parenthood, and it was like we were meeting for the first time, family to family.

I had wondered before our meeting if West—six months old—would display a special connection to Daniel, if there really was some magic carried in their shared DNA, if our son would recognize him, cling to him, fall asleep against his chest. But he didn't. West greeted him with joyful curiosity, the same way he greeted any stranger, and then returned to my arms to nurse once again.

Several months after we met Rebecca and Daniel at the pizza place, Kellie and I drove six hours across the state—baby tucked in his infant car seat in the back—to meet them again in their new home.

The fog of new parenthood had lifted, so the ease between us was instant this time. Rebecca and I each claimed a spot at her kitchen table, sat with coffee, and watched as our children chewed on toys and pulled themselves across the wood floors. Conversation between us was continuous. We found a rhythm of interrupting one thought with another, then picking up where we left off, all the while tending to babies as needed— rising to lift and nurse them, change a diaper, or pull a board book from a mouth. At one point we loaded my infant car seat into Rebecca's car, and our babies rode side by side in the back, Rebecca and me side by side in the front, so that we could drive into town for coffee. Something about going out for coffee with a friend, and about having companionship from beginning to end, felt at once frivolous and necessary. Time with Rebecca was a respite from the solitude and repetition of early motherhood, a dose of medicine I needed.

Kellie and Daniel found their places just as easily. They spent their time rewiring Daniel's carpentry studio, or salvaging beams from a nearby teardown, or driving to the forest to cut up fallen trees for firewood.

We became parallel, symbiotic. Two families on either side of the state. Sometimes they traveled to us; other times we traveled to them. Our boys knew and remembered each other. They splashed each other in an outdoor tub, climbed trees that had grown sideways over the shore of Puget Sound, built forts together out of cardboard.

The beauty of our new extended family had little to do with anything we had asked for or planned. We had begun only with what we had sensed was a rapport between us. We had agreed only to stay in some kind of loose touch over the years.

And yet we wound up with something I'd never quite had and never would have thought to plan for. I'd grown up with cousins, but none were my own age. They were five years older, or twelve years older, or three years younger, or twenty years younger. They were also scattered far and wide across the country. My brother was seven years younger than me, and my half siblings were so much older that they were almost like aunts and an uncle.

Now there was something deeply healing to me about having an extended family that was at once chosen but also tied by blood.

Or was it even blood that tied us? In theory, we wanted to know Daniel forever because questions might arise about the

DNA he'd shared with us. We might someday need to ask him about some rare disease or mental illness, to probe beyond the brief set of questions we'd asked over dinner that first night we met.

And then there was the way we'd been trained to see blood as a legitimizing factor, trained to understand that blood equals family. Like many queer families, Kellie and I, while challenging this notion, unconsciously embraced it. Daniel was blood-tied to our child, and therefore he was kin.

But, even more than blood, it was fate that tied us. It was like that film cliché where one stranger saves another's life and they are therefore bound to each other forever. Rebecca and Daniel had agreed to help us build a family, and their choice had a moral weight. Gratitude would forever bind me to them. The love that I felt for West contained a love for them. I couldn't imagine it any other way.

So it made sense to me when, four years after we'd first shared a meal and talked about becoming family, three years after our sons were born, Rebecca called us to ask if we'd considered having another baby. We had.

It was Kellie who, when West turned three, started asking me about a second child. "I don't know," I told her. "You might have to talk me into it." I hoped she would. I wanted my child to grow up with a sibling, but I felt no sense of urgency. If a second child had required us to choose a donor from a sperm bank catalog, I felt certain we wouldn't have even considered it.

"Do you guys want to get pregnant again?" Rebecca asked me that day on the phone. "Because, you know, we are."

It was spring then and, because I was training for a marathon, I suggested that we start trying in August. "No," Kellie said. "It could take years again." I knew she was right. We went to visit them two weeks later.

We conceived on the first try.

Rebecca delivered a second son, Ryan, in November. I delivered a second son, Cedar, in January.

In her book *Recreating Motherhood*, Barbara Katz Rothman writes that the value our society places on genetic relationships is inherently patriarchal, tied to our initial false belief—Aristotle's "flower-pot theory"—that men were the sole genetic contributors. Because the child was of the man, he belonged to the man. Once we recognized that mothers contribute half of the genetic material, we began to see mother and father as having equal claim to their child. Rothman asserts that this is still an inherently patriarchal position, one in which blood ties indicate a kind of ownership, and one in which the work of nurturance is not accounted for.[36] For instance, a man who helps conceive a child via a one-night stand can disappear before the child is born and then resurface years later and claim parental rights.

In our own contemporary culture, we may sometimes act as though we value nurture over nature. These days, I see the truism "love is love" everywhere I turn—on signs, in social media, spoken aloud by celebrities and friends. The statement suggests that love is fundamental, and that factors like gender, race, or age are unimportant, and that love alone is the element that legitimizes a couple or a family. When speaking of adoptees, we've learned to be careful, to use terms like *birth mother* instead of *real mother*, acknowledging that genes and gestation are not the only thing that make a parent "real."

Still, we track our ancestry and meet new genetic relatives—strangers whom we've been told are family—through services like 23andMe. We marvel at the overlapping traits and mannerisms of close relatives raised apart from one another. And when someone does say "real mother," we know exactly what they mean.

"Kellie's not your *real* mom," a neighbor kid once told West, who stood there agape because he had not yet thought to wonder too hard about his origins. At the time, he already understood that his family was different. When other people asked about his father, he had learned to explain, "I have two moms." But as far as I could tell, this was the first moment someone had invited him to wonder about the actual legitimacy of his family—its realness.

———————

Rebecca and I are tied by blood tangentially, but not directly. Our children are blood relatives. She and I are not. Still, she feels more like family than many of my actual blood relations. Rebecca's sister and nieces feel like family, too, though their ties to me have little to do with blood. Rebecca's sister's children have olive skin and the dark eyes they inherited from their father. They bear no resemblance to my own children. I've met Rebecca's mom more times than I can count, and she always hugs me and says my first name sweetly. She knows about what ties us, and so she feels tied to me too.

Meanwhile, Daniel's family of origin is a mystery to me. I see pictures of his relatives on Facebook and have to remind myself that his kin are also my children's blood kin. My children's faces may grow to bear resemblance to the faces I see in photos: the long jawline, the aquiline nose. Or, pieces of these relatives' histories may give clues to my own children's futures—special talents and obsessions, illnesses and struggles. Even when I remind myself of this, it feels distant, hard to reach.

Kin: Your mother who birthed and nursed you, your father who bore witness to your childhood. Your grandmother who let you sleep beside her in the bed when you came to visit. Your aunt who drove you to her home for long weekends, where you lay alongside her golden retriever and looked at the forest through her windows.

Kin: The grandfather you never met who was a ne'er-do-well, whose legacy is a stack of letters and a rainbow painted on a barn in Walla Walla. The uncle who joked around with you in childhood but became distant as you got older. Your second cousin who discovered you online and now sends you a Christmas card every year.

Kin: Your brother who you speak with only a few times a year but carry in your heart. Your aunt by marriage (then lost through divorce) who delighted you with her easy brand of sarcasm.

Kin: The cousins you've only met once or twice in a lifetime. When you see photos of them, some of them look like people you might easily know. Others look like strangers, like someone you might pass in a grocery store and immediately forget.

———

Kellie told me once that she hesitates sometimes when telling our kids about her family's history. It's not quite clear to her: Is her history their history, or is it something else? Long before she spoke this aloud to me, the same question hung in my mind. Does her history matter to our kids because it's their mother's history, or because it is, somehow, their own?

When I look at my own ancestral family photos, I feel like I am looking for clues to who I am, traces of a self that predates me. Are these connections real, I wonder, or are they mythological? Why does ancestral connection hold a sense of magic? Why do I look so hard to find my reflection in blood kin, as if seeing myself in my ancestors will somehow legitimize me?

And yet it turns out that some of my ancestors are not related to me genetically any more than Kellie is genetically related to our sons. Over the course of generations, our genetic ties to individual ancestors dissolve. Geneticist Graham Coop writes that if you trace your genetic heritage, after seven generations "many of your ancestors make no major genetic contribution to you." In other words, your cells carry no significant trace of their DNA. They are no longer your genetic relatives, and yet they are still, of course, your ancestors. Dr. Coop writes, "Genetics is not genealogy."[37]

What if, beyond heredity, families are really a collection of stories, some of them spoken, some of them withheld? Kellie's ancestors were pioneers. My boys spent the first years of their lives in a house that her grandfather and great-grandfather built together. Kellie spends most of her free time splitting wood, building fences and sheds, capturing bee swarms. Cedar can now spot a swarm from a great distance. West is learning to measure wood and use a chop saw. They may one day raise their own families on the same land they were raised on. They may add new walls, new buildings, new fixtures. They do not require Kellie's genes to carry on her legacy.

Four years after West was born, he asked me about where he came from. It was early afternoon on a bright summer day in the wilderness and Cedar—a baby—was on a walk with Kellie, strapped against her chest. That afternoon, West and I were inside our cabin, with light streaming through the windows and making patches on the floor.

I can't remember how the topic came up, but for the first time, I asked him if he wanted to know who his donor was. "Do you want to guess?" I asked him. I was curious if he already had a sense.

"JoAnn?" he said, and I laughed.

"The person who helped us is a man," I said.

"Oh, right," he said. He thought some more and guessed some more, until I finally told him.

"It's Daniel," I said. "Wren's dad."

I watched him closely to see how he'd respond, but I detected neither joy nor surprise nor disappointment.

"Did Daniel help make Cedar too?"

"Yes," I said.

A smile unfurled. It didn't surprise me that this was the thing that mattered to him—that he and his brother had the same origin story, that he wasn't alone in the world.

———

Often, we seem to understand our DNA as a simple blueprint for who we are and what we might become. We see experience as the tool that can push a person toward or away from their full potential, yet we see the potential itself as innate and fixed.

But in truth, DNA and experience interact with each other. The field of epigenetics tells us that genes are turned on and off by experience, that the food we consume, the air we breathe, and how we are nurtured helps determine which genes are expressed and which ones are repressed. Our DNA coding isn't static. For instance, drinking green tea may help regulate the genes that suppress tumors. A sudden loss may trigger depression. And the amount of nurturing and physical contact a child received in the early years may help determine whether or not he'll suffer from anxiety as an adult. Currently, researchers are investigating to what degree trauma in one person's experience can cause a change in DNA that is transmitted from one generation to the next. Experience can become a legacy carried in the blood.

Frances Champagne, a psychologist and genetic researcher, writes that "tactile interaction," physical contact between parent and child, "is so important for the developing brain." Her research shows that "the quality of the early-life environment can change the activity of genes, thus illustrating the dynamic interplay between genes and environmental experiences in shaping development."[38]

When Kellie held our newborn sons against her chest, when she bounced them and rocked them until they slept, she was not simply soothing them in the moment. She was helping to program their DNA, contributing to their genetic legacy. Parents, through the way they nurture, contribute to the child's nature. There is no clear line between the two.

———

What if a partner plays the father role, but she is not a father? What if she's the secondary caregiver, but not the seed-giver? How do we define her? What do we call her?

It takes labor and intention to bond with children you didn't bear. It takes time of holding, bottle-feeding. Children, hungry for the parent they know, resist it—sometimes a little, sometimes a lot. This is the work that many dads must do if they want something approaching equal partnership. But dads also have the luxury of not doing the work and still, always and forever, maintaining the title of Dad.

Kellie doesn't have an automatic title. In the law's eyes, she didn't have an automatic standing—we had to pay a lawyer and fill out endless paperwork for that, because fatherhood defaulted to Daniel. It was his right to keep it; we trusted him to sign it away.

If we could call Kellie *Dad*, without hesitation or irony, her role would be easier to define, because *Dad* is such a flexible role. *Dad* can do barely any of the caretaking, or most of the caretaking, or anything in the middle.

Kellie does all of the mowing and the gutter cleaning and the home repair, but not so much of the bedtime-readying, the bathing, the homework-nagging. Kellie watches movies with the kids on her lap and sometimes takes them on a ride in the tractor. Kellie doesn't really make dinner. If you're going out, it's best to leave a box of tomato soup on the counter and tell her there are hot dogs in the fridge. As a dad, Kellie makes perfect sense.

But we can't—or we won't—call Kellie *Dad*.

It feels better to live with the incongruity of the word *mom*. We're both Mom. She's Mommy Kellie; I'm Mommy Jenn. It's a solution that has always made sense to me. I grew up with Aunt Lauren, Aunt Judy, Aunt Christina, and Aunt Isabel; with Grandma Smith and Grandma Gault. When you have more than one of any given relative, you just add their name at the end.

On a regular basis, Kellie gets called *sir* for being a tall woman in work clothes and a cap. She hates it. In those moments she feels unseen, erased, made into something she's not. Kellie is emphatically a woman. She's a woman emphatic that *woman* should be a term broad enough to include her.

And so we use the word *mom*, needing that term, too, to be large and pliant, to do the work of including moms like her.

In the end, what is family but a collection of disparate parts, assembled as one whole—an electrician and an English teacher, two boys, two dogs, blood grandparents and stepgrandparents, distant cousins, close cousins, aunts and uncles, a donor family, and some permanent friends. The collective whole adds up to something greater than the sum of its parts.

I think of our cabin, assembled by so many hands. I think about me and Laura on our knees laying out the shiplap floor, while Dee followed us with the nail gun. I think of the metal flashing Kellie installed below the roofline to cover up the holes a woodpecker had pecked in our siding. I think about the pine table we bought in the secondhand shop in town.

I think about the imperfections that make the cabin what it

is: the dent in the floor from when I dropped a pan, the scratches from our dogs at play. I think about the paneling on the south side of the loft and how Kellie and Dee argued passionately about whether or not the grain of each board needed to orient in the same direction, and how they were grumpy until the sun set, and we drank beers and finally ate some food and laughed. I think of the knots in the wood that look like bears or ghosts, depending on the angle.

I think about the view just outside the cabin—the mullein that grows taller than me, and the quaking aspen leaves that shimmer, and the downy woodpeckers that pull the beetles from the dying trees. I think about the bluebird house that one year had a long, curly piece of dried grass sticking out of the entrance, blowing the wind like a streamer.

I think about the small closet I built to cover the hot water tank, how Kellie taught me what to measure and how to cut. "You can say you built this," Kellie told me as she lined the first plank along the chop saw which we'd set up on sawhorses outside on the sunny driveway. I think about how love sometimes means that we become each other just a little, Kellie's wide hand on my narrow hand.

A friend of ours once stayed at the cabin without us, and when we returned, we kept finding wallet-size portraits of her. We'd open the silverware drawer, and there she'd be, smiling. I'd check my reflection in the small mirror by the door, and there she'd be again. West asked, "Who's this?" when he found her among his building blocks. It was a good joke, one that lifted my heart, and so we left them there. She also left a small note above the sink, and we left that there too, a declaration that would become part of the walls of this home:

This Place Is All Love,
Merci.

EPILOGUE

It's Thanksgiving weekend, and we're sharing our cabin with Rebecca and Daniel.

There's a giant tub of Duplo blocks on the hardwood floor that's been in use since the moment we all arrived. West and Wren, our four-year-old sons, keep assembling them into buildings and robots, taking them apart, and then starting again from scratch. Daniel and Kellie spend most of the day outside, splitting firewood and stacking it, making piles of fallen branches that we will burn someday.

Rebecca and I stay inside. We both have, in addition to the four-year-olds, babies who require our constant care. Her son Ryan just turned one. He grabs apple slices and crackers from the table, toddles around, disassembles Duplo towers, comes back and pulls on Rebecca's shirt. My own second child, Cedar, is nine months old. He doesn't walk yet, but he adds to the chaos by crawling over to the dog beds and rolling around where they've left their hair and debris. He is constantly drooling and puts the Duplos in his mouth.

In the evening, when the sun goes down over the hills, Daniel and Kellie come inside. The fire in the woodstove blazes—it's so hot inside, I've cracked a couple of windows. Yesterday was Thanksgiving Day, and we spent it on the road. Dinner was tacos on a paper plate, purchased from the food truck in town. Today we've got a chicken in the oven and potatoes on the stove. We've got whiskey to add to warm cider and a bottle of red wine. We've got kale salad with pomegranate seeds just so we can throw something green on a plate. We've got more than we need. Our table was made for four, so we eat with the babies on our laps. When they get restless, we nurse them on the left side and continue to hold our forks with our right hands. We let West and Wren continue to play Duplos because, miraculously, they are still quiet and happy.

It seems foolhardy to squeeze two families of four into a single cabin in the middle of winter, but somehow it works. After dinner, Rebecca, Daniel, and Wren climb the ladder to the loft. Daniel reaches back down and Kellie passes them their baby, Ryan. Downstairs, Kellie reads to West in one twin bed, while I nurse Cedar to sleep in the other. Twenty minutes later, the lights are out, and the cabin is quiet. It's only eight thirty, but I fall asleep easily and don't wake until morning.

After breakfast the next day, I load Cedar in the front pack and bundle West in his coat and mittens. Kellie and Daniel are already starting a chainsaw, cutting up aspen trees that dried up and fell. Rebecca is reading to her kids. Outside, the sun has just crested the hill; it lights up the tips of yellow grass on the patch of land we are walking through. The path is steep. As we climb it, heading toward the larger dirt road, West lags behind. I stop and turn around. I wait for him to catch up. "My legs are tired," he says. "You can do it," I say. "Remember that rock at the top of the hill? You can climb it when we get there." He starts trudging again, one boot in front of the other.

I remember standing in this same spot six years ago at the end of summer. I stood alone then, wishing for a child, wondering if one would ever find its way to me. I remember the feeling of hope—hope, the most desperate, painful thing—blooming like a wound. The me of six years ago wears the same coat and the same shoes that I wear now. She looks at those shoes. She kicks gravel. The cold air stings. I want to reach through time and hand her a picture of this moment: Cedar looks up at me steadily from my front pack carrier. He's got two teeth on top, two on the bottom. He is remarkably strong, this baby, not unlike a monkey: lean and driven by energy.

And then there is West, with the wide brown eyes, who has always been tender. West, who would like to keep me up until midnight most nights, talking, talking, talking. Which is all I ever wanted. One day in the car, just a few months ago, he asked me questions about ghosts from the back seat. Were they real or not real? He wanted to know, and when I gave him an equivocal answer, he asked a million more questions, like, "If they're real, do you think they can touch you?" and "Can something be real and not real at the same time?" *This*, I kept thinking, *is the reason I always wanted children.*

I want the me of six years ago to glimpse me now, just for one brief instant, to see West in his navy blue boots with the bright orange soles, to see that I wait for him, that he arrives and takes my hand, and that we walk together.

I want to whisper in her ear that if it had been easy to conceive, then the cabin down the hill would be empty right now. Kellie would be chainsawing alone, and there would be no giant box of Duplos, no half brothers to run around with. I would likely have one child, not two, and that child would not be West.

Or, if it had been harder to conceive, the me of six years ago might be standing here now, same shoes, same coat, kicking gravel. She might have given up on having children and given herself more deeply to solitude. She might have written several books by now, or qualified for the Boston Marathon, or given herself to some project unimaginable to the living, breathing me that's here on this path today.

But the life I have now, the one I've landed in, is the one where I have more family than I asked for, more than I ever thought to dream of. That we could ask for such a thing—that one evening at dinner we could ask two near-strangers if they'd join our lives forever, that they could say yes and mean it, that we could find ourselves here years later—astounds me. It will always astound me.

When you break the contract of cisgender heterosexuality, you depart from the social expectations of marriage, of children, of gender, and you risk losing family members who may reject you. You are essentially, in the moment of coming out, alone in the world, hanging your life on a single truth about yourself.

It never stops feeling that way. Even if you are lucky, even if your closest family members accept you without hesitation, you may not be able to shake the feeling that your place in the larger family is tenuous. At Thanksgiving, at graduations, at family reunions, you will have to assess how much you can say and to whom. Who knows and who doesn't? Who will flinch if you utter the words "my partner?" And always, you might wonder how your parents really feel about who you've turned out to be.

It's a fundamentally queer principle to build a family out of the pieces you have, to pick and choose what stays and what goes. Queers have always defined family differently than the culture at large. We've always needed to reach beyond our blood kin, to draw close those who know the pain of our particular difference and those who see us.

When I was a fifth grader who was worried she might be gay, the life I pictured was a lonely one: a life of pining, of sleeping alone, of shutting myself inside, not just loverless but friendless too.

I had never imagined that being queer could mean the

opposite—that my world would grow larger to compensate for the ways it had grown smaller, that there would be Dr. Normans, yes, but there would also be Rebeccas and Daniels—people willing to tie their lives to ours to help us reach our goal. I had never imagined that being queer could mean a chance to shed the expectations of tradition, to shed the insularity of heredity and gender, to define family on my own terms and remake everything new.

I had never imagined a life where I could live not just with a partner and two children, but with a sense of connection to a larger community, a knowledge that the love that made our family extended far beyond the walls of our home.

READING GROUP GUIDE

1. Throughout her journey, Jenn learns that family doesn't necessarily mean being related by blood. Think about your own inner circle—who do you consider family?

2. Describe Jenn and Kellie's friends. In what ways do they each help the couple along in their journey?

3. Jenn always knew she was destined to be a parent. What choices have you had to make so far around parenthood?

4. Describe how members of the LGBTQ community found ways to work outside the patriarchal medical system. Can you see any contemporary parallels? How does the queer community—or other marginalized groups—navigate systems that are hostile to them?

5. How did Jenn's upbringing influence her view of parenthood? How did your own childhood shape how you view what it means to be a parent?

6. Jenn's relationship with her mother is a little tense, but ultimately, she sees that she deserves "a seat at the table." Who sits around your proverbial table? Did you have to come to terms with any past tension before they were welcome there?

7. Think about the challenges that Jenn faces throughout her story. Can you relate to any of them? Are there any you hadn't thought about before?

8. The history of gynecology, artificial insemination, and sperm banks is very ethically fraught. How does that shape your impression of contemporary fertility treatment?

9. Initially Jenn is happy to pick a sperm donor from a binder full of strangers, while Kellie wants to have a personal relationship with their donor. Which method would you prefer, and why?

10. Throughout Jenn's story, she often confronts the belief that a family should consist of a straight, cisgender couple and their biological children. How did she react to that prejudice? How can we work to make the concept of parenthood and family inclusive to all?

A CONVERSATION
WITH THE AUTHOR

What inspired you to write *The Other Mothers?*

As I was living through this story, I found myself surprised by how many twists and turns my journey was taking and how often the fertility industry disappointed me. When Daniel and Rebecca entered our lives, I was so deeply moved. Their generosity changed something in me and my perception of community, and this made me want to tell the story. It's a funny thing, because many queer parents don't want to be asked—especially by strangers or acquaintances—how they made their families. The experience of building a family is deeply private, not something people want to share with anyone and everyone. And yet, at the same time, for me personally, it's something I want to talk about.

You've written several essays for a variety of online and print outlets. Did you find that your writing process changed when tackling a bigger project?

Yes! I had already started writing this book when I began writing and publishing shorter pieces. In part, I wrote those shorter pieces because I really needed the sense of gratification that came with actually finishing something and then sending it out in the world. It gave me the confidence I needed to keep working on the book, which went through many drafts and iterations. But eventually, the shorter essays became a distraction, and I had to quit writing them to focus solely on the book.

What books do you have on your bedside table right now?
Well, it's summer right now, and I've been enjoying the chance to catch up on some great novels. I'm currently reading *An American Marriage* by Tayari Jones, which is so incredibly compelling, and just finished *Little Fires Everywhere* by Celeste Ng. I also just finished listening to Kim Gordon read her memoir *Girl in a Band*, which gave me a fun window into various New York art and rock scenes as I was doing my very rural domestic tasks like weeding the garden or feeding the chickens.

What's it like knowing that you've walked in the footsteps of a long line of LGBTQ+ people who fought to become parents?
I feel grateful for their radicalism and innovation. By the time I came out as a lesbian (in the '90s), I knew that parenting would be an option for me, and this is because of a lineage of people who fought battles on many fronts: feminists who worked for

fair access to reproductive education and care, communities of queer people who built networks to facilitate inseminations, and those who fought legal battles to protect families. Many of those protections are still fragile, and—as I hope this book shows—we still have plenty of work to do to become a culture that truly supports LGBTQ+ people who decide to be parents. I think I sometimes fall into the trap of imagining social progress as a straight line, but the people I talked to were part of incredibly radical active communities that no longer exist in the same way. They brought a kind of vision and determination to their lives that I admire and hope to learn from.

What did your research process look like?

The research was the very last layer I added to the book, and it changed my understanding of my own story. It started with me reaching out to the lesbians in my community who had conceived in the generation before me, and so I wound up doing a lot of one-on-one interviews. This was the very human and community-oriented side of my research process. It fed me.

At the same time, I read a lot books and articles about the history of the assisted reproduction. Though my personal experience with the fertility industry felt like an experience with patriarchy and paternalism, I hadn't yet directly connected my experience to the roots of the industry. But once I started doing the research a funny thing happened. Any research question I asked yielded an immediate and clear connection to patriarchy.

For instance, I'd decide that I should look into the first known insemination, and it wouldn't take me long to discover that it had been done without the patient's consent. I'd get curious about the history of the speculum, and learn that it was developed by Marion J. Sims, who I already had a passing awareness of for his exploitation of and violent abuse of enslaved women. The more research I conducted, the clearer it became that the fertility industry is deeply tied to sexist, racist, and heteronormative ideals.

A memoir is a very personal piece of work—were there any parts that you found difficult to write?

What I found most difficult was writing about my family of origin. My relationship to each of my parents and my experience of childhood felt relevant to the main storyline, but I found it hard to decide what aspects of that story needed to go in the book, and what might be better saved for another piece of writing. I spent plenty of time writing, cutting, rewriting, and then recutting.

What advice would you give to anyone out there who's still on the hard path to parenthood?

One of the things that I found most challenging throughout my journey was that people were always offering me unsolicited advice, so mainly I want to validate the experience of people on that path: it is hard to be in limbo, and—if you are in a stage where you are trying to conceive—hard to maintain a positive relationship with your body when it isn't doing what you're asking of it. It's easy to begin to see each missed attempt as some kind of personal failure. But you are not a failure, and your ability or inability to get pregnant is not a reflection of your worth.

Also, more generally, I would say that the whole process—from if and when and how to become parents, or responding to a surprise pregnancy, or waiting for an adoption—it's all rife with uncertainty, and I think that that's our initiation into parenting. Before I was a parent, I imagined I would have all kinds of control over what my family life would look like, but it turns out I don't! My children are their own people with their own strong wills. I think a lot of parenting is relinquishing the illusion that you control your life.

West's question, "Can something be real and not-real at the same time?" is simultaneously adorable and poignant... Can you leave us with any other pieces of kid-wisdom?

Well, I can tell you about something Cedar said the other day that really blew me out of the water. We were reading a graphic novel called *Cardboard*, and in one scene a neighbor offers a plate of freshly baked cookies to the protagonist, who is a widower. He turns her down, not wanting to give her the "wrong idea," and I wasn't sure if Cedar (who is seven now) would understand the romantic subtext, so I asked him, "Do you know why he keeps saying no to her?" Without missing a beat, he said, "It's because he doesn't like himself very much." In that moment, he explained to me something I had been trying to figure out in my own life, i.e. why some people actively distance themselves from people who are kind to them.

RESOURCES

The Sperm Bank of California
https://www.thespermbankofca.org

MAIA Midwifery & Fertility, specializing in LGBTQ family-building
http://maiamidwifery.com

Family Equality Council
https://www.familyequality.org

Lambda Legal
https://www.lambdalegal.org

Movement Advancement Project: Maps of LGBTQ equality by state
https://www.lgbtmap.org/equality-maps

Human Rights Campaign: Adoption Options Overview
https://www.hrc.org/resources/
adoption-options-overview

GLAD: Standards for LGBT Families
https://www.glad.org/protecting-families/p4

Trans and Gender Diverse Parents Guide
https://www.rainbowfamilies.com.au/
trans_and_gender_diverse_parents_guide_released

Children of Lesbians and Gays Everywhere (COLAGE)
https://www.colage.org

Donor Sibling Registry
https://donorsiblingregistry.com

NOTES

1   Robert Edwards and Patrick Steptoe, *A Matter of Life: The Story of IVF—a Medical Breakthrough* (London: Hutchinson, 1980), Kindle.

2   Kate Brian, "The Amazing Story of IVF: 35 Years and 5 Million Babies Later," *The Guardian*, July 12, 2013, https://www.theguardian.com/society/2013/jul/12/story-ivf-five-million-babies.

3   Edwards and Steptoe, *A Matter of Life*.

4   Melinda Spohn, "Risking Pregnancy for 'Mr. Right': Unintended Pregnancy and Female Mating Preferences," *Journal of Evolutionary Psychology* 29, no. 1–2 (October 2006), https://www.questia.com/library/journal/1G1-155027151/risking-pregnancy-for-mr-right-unintended-pregnancy.

5   Jenny A. Higgins, "Pregnancy Ambivalence and Long-Acting Reversible Contraceptive (LARC) Use among Young Adult Women: A Qualitative Study," *Perspectives on Sexual & Reproductive Health* 49, no. 3 (September 2017): 149–156. doi:10.1363/psrh.12025.

6   Gretchen Livingston and D'Vera Cohn, "The New Demography of American Motherhood," Pew Research Center, May 6, 2010, https://www

.pewsocialtrends.org/2010/05/06/the-new-demography-of-american
-motherhood/.

7   Sonia Fader, "Sperm Banking History," California Cryobank,
accessed February 2, 2020, https://www.cryobank.com/learning-center
/sperm-banking-101/sperm-banking-history/.

8   "Pat Shively," accessed February 2, 2020, http://ladyfest.org
/LadiesWeLike/Shively_Pat.html.

9   Allison Wolfe, "Pat Shively: Women's Health Care Pioneer," *Ampersand*,
May 6, 2016, http://www.ampersandla.com/pat-shively-womens-health-care
-pioneer/.

10   David Plotz, *The Genius Factory: The Curious History of the Nobel Prize
Sperm Bank* (New York: Random House, 2006).

11   Robert Klark Graham, *The Future of Man* (North Quincy, MA:
Christopher Publishing House, 1970).

12   Lori B. Andrews, *The Clone Age* (New York: Henry Holt and Company,
1999).

13   Alix Spiegel, "FDA Advises Sperm Banks on Gay Donors," *Day to
Day*, NPR, May 17, 2005, https://www.npr.org/templates/story/story
.php?storyId=4655231.

14   Amy Agigian, *Baby Steps* (Middletown, CT: Wesleyan University Press,
2004).

15   Rene Almeling, *Sex Cells: The Medical Market for Eggs and Sperm*
(Berkeley: University of California Press, 2011).

16   A.D. Hard, "Artificial Impregnation," *The Medical
World* 27 (1909): 163–164, https://babel.hathitrust.org/cgi
/pt?id=mdp.39015026093826&view=1up&seq=177.

17 John Seabrook, "The Last Babylift," *The New Yorker*, May 3, 2010, https://www.newyorker.com/magazine/2010/05/10/the-last-babylift.

18 "A Critique of Bertha and Harry Holt's Work While Setting up Intercountry Adoption in South Korea," *Transracialeyes* (blog), August 11, 2011, https://transracialeyes.wordpress.com/2011/08/11/a-brief-historical -overview-of-the-life-and-times-of-harry-and-bertha-holt-and-the-origin-of -international-adoption/.

19 "A Critique of Bertha and Harry Holt…".

20 Joanne Lee, "The Holt Adoption Agency: Changing the Face of America's Social and Ethnic Relations," accessed February 8, 2020, http://www .dartmouth.edu/~hist32/History/S29%20-%20Holt%20Agency.htm.

21 Harry Holt, "Harry Holt's 'Dear Friends' Letter," 1955, The Adoption History Project, February 24, 2012, https://darkwing.uoregon .edu/~adoption/archive/HoltDearFriendsltr.htm/.

22 United Nations Commission on Human Rights, *Report of the Special Rapporteur on the Sale of Children, Child Prostitution and Child Pornography*, January 27, 2000, https://www.refworld.org/publisher,UNCHR,,GTM,,,0 .html.

23 Sharon LaFraniere, "Chinese Officials Seized and Sold Babies, Parents Say," *New York Times*, August 4, 2011, https://www.nytimes.com/2011/08/05 /world/asia/05kidnapping.html?_r=1&scp=1&sq=longhui&st=cse.

24 David M. Smolin, "Child Laundering: How the Intercountry Adoption System Incentivizes the Practices of Buying, Trafficking, and Stealing Children," *The Wayne Law Review* 52, no. 1 (2006): 113–159, http://citeseerx.ist.psu .edu/viewdoc/download?doi=10.1.1.693.3159&rep=rep1&type=pdf.

25 Dr. Jane Aronson, "The Trouble with International Adoption Is Not

Trafficking: It's the Global Orphan Crisis," *HuffPost*, September 20, 2011, https://www.huffpost.com/entry/the-trouble-with-internat_b_971226.

26 "Foster and Adoption Laws," Movement Advancement Project, February 7, 2020, http://www.lgbtmap.org/equality-maps/foster_and_adoption_laws.

27 J. Marion Sims, *The Story of My Life* (New York: D. Appleton and Co., 1884), https://archive.org/details/storyofmylif00sims/page/n4/mode/2up.

28 Sims, *The Story of My Life*.

29 Rose Eveleth, "Why No One Can Design a Better Speculum," *The Atlantic*, November 17, 2014, https://www.theatlantic.com/health/archive/2014/11/why-no-one-can-design-a-better-speculum/382534/.

30 Judith P. Rooks, CNM, MPH, MS, "The History of Midwifery," *Our Bodies Ourselves*, May 30, 2012, https://www.ourbodiesourselves.org/book-excerpts/health-article/history-of-midwifery/.

31 Hannah Dahlen, "Episiotomy during Childbirth: Not Just a 'Little Snip,'" *The Conversation*, January 14, 2015, https://theconversation.com/episiotomy-during-childbirth-not-just-a-little-snip-36062.

32 Racial and Ethnic Disparities Continue in Pregnancy-Related Deaths," Centers for Disease Control and Prevention, September 5, 2019, https://www.cdc.gov/media/releases/2019/p0905-racial-ethnic-disparities-pregnancy-deaths.html.

33 Danielle Braff, "Here's Why Many Black Women Are Silent about Their Struggle with Infertility," *Chicago Tribune*, June 29, 2019, https://www.chicagotribune.com/lifestyles/sc-fam-black-women-fertility-20190629-udbld2hkpnexfofxg325ajshr4-story.html.

34 Elizabeth A. Harris, "Same-Sex Parents Still Face Legal Complications," *New York Times*, June 20, 2017, https://www.nytimes.com/2017/06/20/us/gay-pride-lgbtq-same-sex-parents.html.

35 J. Kremer, "The Haematogenous Reproduction Theory of Aristotle," *Ned Tijdschr Geneeskd* 147, no. 51 (2003): https://www.ncbi.nlm.nih.gov /pubmed/14735853.

36 Barbara Katz Rothman, *Recreating Motherhood* (New Jersey: Rutgers University Press, 2000).

37 Dr. Graham Coop (@Graham_Coop), Twitter post, October 16, 2018, https://twitter.com/Graham_Coop/status/1052307076184035328.

38 Kathryn M.A. Gudsnuk and Frances A. Champagne, "Epigenetic Effects of Early Developmental Experiences," *Clinics in Perinatology* 38, no. 4 (December 2011): 703–717, doi.org/10.1016/j.clp.2011.08.005.

ACKNOWLEDGMENTS

It took me years to write this book while parenting young children and working, and I'm grateful for all of the people who helped keep me on the path.

Thanks to Dee Williams, whose diligent work and collaboration on *The Big Tiny* helped me learn how to build a frame for my own story. Thanks to Elissa Wald and Stephanie Andersen for valuable feedback on early drafts, along with Lynn Shattuck, Susan Moshovsky, Becki Kapelusznik, and Alexis Wolff, who provided inspiration at a time when I so desperately needed it. Thanks to Samantha Dunn and the Writing by Writers program for giving this project a push, and also for the days of good food and conversation.

Thanks to my agent, Rachel Vogel, for her steadfastness. Thanks to Anna Michels and Jenna Jankowski for their vision, insight, and belief in this project. Thanks to Manu Velasco for their keen eye. Thanks to Cheri Lucas Rowlands at Longreads for her edits to the chapter "Becoming Family." Thanks to Artist Trust for financial support.

Thanks to those in my community who so generously shared their time and information with me: Michi Thacker, Audrey Daye, Jan Shafer, Carolyn Skye, Helen J. Thornton, and Joyce. Thanks to Sherron Mills, Alice Ruby, and Kristin Kali for helping me understand the industry, past and present. Thanks to Shelbi Day for her expertise in LGBTQ adoption access.

Thanks to the writers in my daily life who keep me in the work: Kathleen Byrd, Sarah Tavis, Anne DeMarcken, Marilyn Freeman, Jen Cerasoli, El Lee, and Irene Keliher.

Thanks to my family of origin: to my parents for their interest and candor, and to my siblings for being a steady presence and welcome diversion.

Thanks to my chosen family and network: JoAnn, Kathy, RJ, Irina, Katy, Vic, Dave, Stella, Ruby, Jen W., Carlin, Jennifer C., Jerry, Richard, Ron Sr. and Ron Jr., Rebecca and Daniel and all their kin.

Special thanks to Kellie, West, and Cedar for sharing this life with me.

ABOUT THE AUTHOR

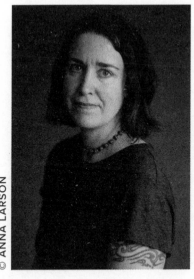

Jennifer Berney's essays have appeared in *Longreads*, *Tin House*, *The Offing*, *The New York Times*, *The Washington Post*, and many other publications. Jennifer holds an MFA in Creative Writing from The University of Washington. She lives with her partner and two children in the Pacific Northwest. *The Other Mothers* is her first book.